NATURAL MEDICINE

for

Heart Disease

The Best Alternative Methods for Prevention and Treatment

- *High Cholesterol*
- *High Blood Pressure*
- *Stroke*
- *Chest Pain*
- *Other Circulatory Problems*

GLENN S. ROTHFELD, M.D.

AND SUZANNE LeVERT

RODALE

Rodale Press, Inc.
Emmaus, Pennsylvania

This book is intended as a reference volume only, not as a medical manual. The information given here is designed to help you make informed decisions about your health. It is not intended as a substitute for any treatment that may have been prescribed by your doctor. If you suspect that you have a medical problem, we urge you to seek competent medical help.

Library of Congress Cataloging-in-Publication Data

    Rothfeld, Glenn.
        Natural medicine for heart disease : the best alternative methods
    for prevention and treatment / Glenn Rothfeld, with Suzanne LeVert.
        p.   cm.
    Includes index.
        ISBN 0–87596–289–0 paperback
        1. Heart—Diseases—Alternative treatment. 2. Heart—Diseases—
    Prevention. I. LeVert, Suzanne. II Title.
    RC684.A48R68   1996
    616.1—dc20   95-24445

Distributed in the book trade by St. Martin's Press

2 4 6 8 10 9 7 5 3   paperback

Dedication

....

*To Magi, who holds my heart,
and my daughter, Carly, who warms it*

G. S. R.

Acknowledgments

....

*I would like to thank Madeleine Morel,
Barbara Lowenstein and Rodale Press for their
help in hatching and shepherding this idea;
AMR'TA, makers of IBIS, an extraordinary data base
of natural medicine; Richard Glickman-Simon,
Catherine LeBlanc, Dr. Daren Fan, Loretta Levitz,
Lori Grace, Nancy Lipman and others who
helped me with their comments and encouragement.
I am also grateful to the many patients who
brought me ideas and inspired me with their own
journeys toward better health.*

Contents

"Hearts don't break, they bend and wither."

H. W. Thompson, 1940

Understanding
the Alternatives

1

$\mathcal{F}$orty-eight-year-old Troy Williams,* a lawyer with a public
defenders' office, suffered a mild heart attack just as he was wrapping
up an important case. His wife, Clarissa, called me a few days later
for advice. "I know that Troy is afraid now and wants to do anything
it takes to keep this from happening again and from having to spend
any more time in the hospital," she revealed. I asked Clarissa to have
the hospital forward Troy's records to me and made an appointment
to see her husband the following week.

Troy's records showed that one of his coronary arteries was
almost completely blocked by atherosclerotic plaque and another

*Names have been changed in this and all case histories recounted in this book.
Some case histories are composites based on the experiences of several of my
patients.

artery was on its way to becoming so. Fortunately, his heart attack was minor and Troy had every chance of making a full recovery. If his wife was correct in thinking that her husband was ready to change his lifestyle, Troy had a good chance of reversing the blockage that had already taken place, and he could probably do so without the use of drugs or surgery. Two cardiac drugs, a vasodilator and a calcium-channel blocker to assist blood flow to the heart, were prescribed to him after his heart attack. They could probably be slowly withdrawn as the health of his heart improved.

"What are my options?" Troy asked me when he arrived for his appointment. "My cousin has gone through three balloon angioplasty operations in the last five years. It's cost him a lot of money and worry. He also feels like he's lost control of his life. Can I avoid that?" I told him that it was possible, but that it would take a different kind of commitment than he was used to making: A long-term commitment to healing his body and spirit. He agreed to at least consider the options I could offer him.

I then asked Troy a series of questions that, at first glance, had little to do with the health of his coronary arteries: what he ate on a typical day, how much he drank, if he liked his job, what he did with his time off. We also discussed how the heart attack had made him feel, both emotionally and physically. We talked for almost an hour and I examined him carefully. Then I began to give him my opinion about the best way for him to heal his heart. Based on what he told me, I developed a treatment plan for him involving a low-fat diet, an exercise plan, and a time each day for meditation and self-affirmation.

I also warned him that what I offered was not a quick, and often temporary, fix like a balloon angioplasty. But if he could make substantial changes to his diet, learn new ways to cope with the stresses inherent in his job, and maintain an exercise regimen, the benefits to his whole self—his mind, spirit and body—would be both long-lasting and extend far beyond his artery walls. In addition, I told him that there were other systems of healing, including those developed in India and China, that he might want to explore on his own.

With Clarissa's help, Troy began eating a diet deriving just 15 percent of its calories from fat (less than half the fat of his previous diet, and of the diet most Americans eat). The eating plan emphasized green leafy vegetables for their mineral content and fiber. He also began taking supplements of vitamin C, magnesium, L-carnitine, and essential fatty acids, as well as half an aspirin tablet each night to thin his blood a bit and make its passage through the vessels easier.

Troy started a gentle exercise program of stretches and yoga postures to increase oxygen to his tissues. After a while, the cardiologist gave Troy the okay to do some aerobic exercise. Troy chose to ride a stationary bike and use a StairMaster; and before he began, we discussed his negative tendency toward goal-oriented behavior. We also talked more about how Troy saw his heart attack as a "chink" in his male armor, and the risk he ran of turning his exercise and diet plan into yet two more opportunities to compete with others—and with himself.

In further meetings, I helped Troy see the need to let go of some of his competitiveness, and we formed "affirmations"—adages and sayings—that he could repeat to himself such as "I don't have to prove how strong I am" and "I feel powerful when I'm relaxed." He meditated for about 20 minutes a day using these affirmations.

Six months after his heart attack, Troy is feeling healthier, stronger, and more optimistic than at any time in the past. He has been relatively consistent about eating a low-fat, high-fiber diet, has performed 20 minutes of meditation every day, and 45 minutes of exercise every other day, and has begun to discuss with his co-workers the need to change what had been a cutthroat environment in the public defenders' office. Troy has also developed an interest in Eastern philosophy and, particularly, Chinese medicine. We are now exploring acupuncture as another treatment option.

Natural prescription: Low-fat diet, aerobic exercise, meditation and self-affirmation.

Heart Disease and Natural Medicine

Heart disease and related conditions like high blood pressure and high cholesterol levels affect more Americans than any other single disease. In recent decades, millions of dollars have been spent developing new diagnostic procedures, new drugs, and new surgical techniques. Although this new technology is responsible for cutting in half the number of people who die from heart attacks and strokes, it has done little either to prevent the disease from occurring in the first place or to restore people to true health.

This has led more and more people like Troy to search for health care solutions that are less expensive, less painful, and longer-lasting. All this is creating a movement away from technology and toward a fuller understanding of how to maintain the balance of body and spirit. This new movement, which is the true essence of health, is developing even among the most conventional medical institutions in this country.

Since you're reading this book, chances are that you, too, are hoping to find a way to heal your heart that helps you avoid (as much as possible) costly hospital visits and pharmacy bills. You may also be searching for a way to cope with some of the underlying reasons why your body is no longer healthy. Fortunately, there are many options available to you that will help you accomplish all of these goals. For the sake of simplicity, we've grouped these options under the general terms natural, holistic, or alternative medicine.

Later in this chapter, you'll learn more about the different alternative therapeutic techniques and philosophies of health that you may want to use to help treat your heart disease. First, however, let's take a look at natural medicine in general.

Why Natural Medicine?

Without doubt, most Americans have been brought up believing that almost anything can be fixed, and fixed quickly. Television programs "prove" it to us every day: All problems are worked out within a half hour or an hour; only the most complicated issues require a two-hour movie or an extended mini-series to resolve. In our medical world, the same mind-set is at work: If your arteries are clogged, bust the plaque right out with a balloon or re-route blood through a by-pass. Take drugs to lower cholesterol levels and/or blood pressure. And if worse comes to worst, you can always trade in your damaged heart for a brand new one.

If drugs and surgery can work so well to keep you up and running, why bother to address the underlying causes of your medical problems or take the time to help the body heal itself? The truth is, of course, that the body is not merely a machine made of interchangeable parts, nor is true health defined merely as being "up and running." Instead, each human body is a unique entity comprising not only organs and tissues but spirit, intellect, and emotion. Health exists when all of these components work in balance with each other and in coordination with the body's natural rhythms and cycles.

To attain health in this sense takes time and commitment, especially in this society where the very habits of daily life often conspire to undermine spiritual and physical well-being. Bringing the body into harmony means providing it with the right kind of fuel by eating properly, massaging its organs and tissues through regular exercise, and allowing its internal environment to rest and regenerate in peace through meditation and other relaxation techniques. When the body falls into a state of imbalance, natural medicine offers its own set of therapeutic agents, such as herbs and essential oils, that come directly from nature and thus are meant to help the body heal itself rather than take over the body's functions.

Without question, there are times when modern medical technology and pharmacology can seem miraculous. Antibiotics fight infections that would otherwise spread through the body too quickly for natural medicine to effectively stop them. The surgical removal of cancerous tissue may be necessary to halt the invasion of abnormal cells into essential organs. And for many people with advanced cardiovascular disease, surgery to unclog coronary arteries or drugs to reduce high blood pressure are the only ways to prevent a fatal heart attack or stroke, at least in the short term.

However, current research is showing that reducing risk factors for heart disease and stroke is the best way to assure a full return to cardiovascular health. Increasing numbers of people are turning to one or more natural methods—ranging from dietary changes and vitamin supplements to more comprehensive systems such as Ayurveda and chiropractic—to guide them through the process of regaining their health.

Here's how holistic, natural medicine stands apart from mainstream, Western medicine:

Safer than pharmacology and surgery. Alternative medicine works by helping the body to heal itself, in essence drawing on the innate wisdom of the body to put itself back into balance. Drugs, on the other hand, work by taking over the body's functions; the body never fully heals, then, but is merely compelled to function with help from an outside source. Moreover, drugs often induce side effects that can be avoided with the use of herbs, oils, and other natural remedies. Surgery, needless to say, is invasive, usually painful, and by nature, often disfiguring.

Focuses on the individual, not the illness. Practitioners of natural medicine recognize that every person with cardiovascular disease developed the condition under a set of circumstances wholly unique to that individual. Because no one cause exists for heart disease, no one type of therapy will cure it. Even with mainstream medicine, it is rare that one simple solution—one drug or one surgical procedure—will cure someone with cardiovascular disease once and for all. Alleviating heart disease naturally, therefore, involves not a simple prescription or operation but a comprehensive plan that takes into consideration the emotional, spiritual, and physical qualities of each individual patient.

Involves the whole body. The heart and blood vessels do not work in isolation from the rest of the body, nor do they remain unaffected by emotions, thoughts, or external stresses. Western medicine, however, tends to look upon organs of the body as separate entities and upon diseases as discrete conditions usually affecting only one or two organs at a time. Most systems of alternative medicine, on the other hand, look at the whole body as a single, unified entity. While a cardiologist concentrates on clearing the coronary arteries of harmful plaque or replacing defective valves, an acupuncturist may locate the source of the problem far from the heart, perhaps in the liver or the spleen.

Validates the emotional component of health. Although it is clear that external stresses and emotional upheavals have a direct impact on the body's ability to function in balance and health, Western medicine has had difficulty in accepting that premise or finding a way to use it to prevent or treat disease. Natural medicine not only acknowledges the integral role our emotions play in maintaining the balance we know as health, but is able to use emotions as *part* of a comprehensive treatment plan for virtually every disease, including heart disease and related conditions.

Preventive, as well as therapeutic. Returning the body to its natural, balanced state is the goal of natural medicine. Many of natural medicine's approaches deal with "disharmony"—the state in which our systems are not functioning effectively. Often, the imbalance has not gone on long enough to show up as illness. Therefore, natural approaches are truly preventive in that they can restore function *before* symptoms appear. In addition, since all symptoms come from the same disharmonies, you might find that other problems, such as headaches or menopausal symptoms, go away when you are treated in a natural way for cardiovascular disease.

Helps you find the natural rhythm of health. Your body is a miraculous system of biochemical actions and reactions that allow you to breathe, digest your food, heal cuts and wounds as well as repair organs after illness, to dream, and to hope. By using natural approaches to restoring and maintaining health, you will be allowing your body to work as nature intended it to without the need for man-made, and potentially side-effect-ridden, pharmaceutical agents.

For these reasons, you may decide to join Troy and millions of other Americans in using one or more natural remedies to help restore your heart and blood vessels to their former state of health. This book is intended to help you sort through the many alternative approaches available and evaluate which ones may work best for your own particular situation.

Nine Natural Approaches

If you're like most Americans who have been diagnosed with heart disease, you are probably taking one or more different drugs. (See Alphabetical Directory of Cardiovascular Drug Groups, pages 210–215, for more information about mainstream drug therapy for heart disease, high blood pressure, and high cholesterol levels.) Before we continue with our discussion about natural remedies for heart disease, it is important to stress that you must *never stop taking medication without first discussing the matter with your physician.*

If you are currently being treated by both a cardiologist or internist and a holistic practitioner, make sure that they both agree that you no longer need to take medication before you stop taking it. Although you may be anxious to forgo the expense and the side effects that stem from many pharmaceutical products, you should be aware that natural medicine works much more slowly and with more subtlety than man-made drugs. Depending on the severity of your heart disease, then, you may need to continue taking your medication for a period of several weeks or months, until the alternative therapy you've chosen has had a chance to effect the changes necessary to return your body to its natural state of balance.

In this book, we explore nine different types of alternative therapy that are appropriate for treating cardiovascular disease. In many ways, they are all interrelated, having in common the aspects of balance and self-healing discussed above and using many of the same therapeutic agents. However, some are more effective than others in the treatment of heart disease and will be covered in more depth.

Our first tier of therapy includes diet and nutrition, exercise, and relaxation techniques. A high-fat diet, sedentary lifestyle, and stress are three of the most serious risk factors for the development of heart disease. We'll show you how to eat, move, and unwind so that your body can restore itself in a natural way.

In addition, you'll learn about six other techniques that you may find helpful in your search for safe and comfortable health care. Each stems from a very different and complicated system of thought and requires much more information than you'll be able to garner from this book. But we'll give you the basic information and, in Chapter 3, help you decide which alternative, or combination of alternatives, suits you best.

In the meantime, here's a brief overview of the alternative therapies for cardiovascular disease discussed in this book:

FIRST-TIER ALTERNATIVES

Nutrition and vitamin therapy. If the phrase "You are what you eat" is a cliché, it is one that has special meaning today. Mainstream physicians, who only recently had discounted the impact of diet on health, are beginning to understand how essential a proper diet is to the overall health of the body. The health of your heart and blood vessels is especially affected by the food you eat. Indeed, a proper diet is the mainstay of any therapy for cardiovascular disease, both mainstream and alternative. Chapter 4 will cover the essentials of a low-fat, high-fiber diet as well as explain the new research confirming what many alternative practitioners have known for years: that certain vitamins and minerals, known as antioxidants, protect your body from disease.

Exercise. In 1992, the American Heart Association added a sedentary lifestyle to its list of top ten risk factors for the development of heart disease. Finally, mainstream medicine formally recognized what had always been an integral component of alternative medicine: that regular exercise helps the body maintain the internal equilibrium and balance we know as health. Exercise helps the intestines digest food more efficiently, the muscles stay strong and lithe, the brain remain alert and stimulated.

No system of the body appears to benefit more from exercise

than the cardiovascular system. All forms of physical activity, from the most passive and relaxing to the most vigorous, help to prevent and reduce both high blood pressure and coronary heart disease. In Chapter 6, you'll learn how exercise benefits the cardiovascular system from both the mainstream and alternative perspectives. You'll also find some tips to help you incorporate regular physical activity into your daily life.

Relaxation and meditation. Your heart and blood vessels react to stress in very physical ways that, over the long haul, can lead to illness. All forms of alternative medicine recognize the importance of reducing the impact of stress on your body and spirit. Moreover, as studies by Dean Ornish, cardiologist and author of *Dr. Dean Ornish's Guide to Reversing Heart Disease*, have shown, understanding and accepting your feelings and emotions about your heart disease and its underlying causes are important steps on your road to recovery. Chapter 7 will guide you through several different relaxation, meditation, and self-affirmation exercises.

SECOND-TIER ALTERNATIVES

Acupuncture. Stemming from a centuries-old system of traditional Chinese medicine, acupuncture views health not only as the absence of disease but as the ability to maintain a balanced and harmonious internal environment. It is based on the view that humanity is part of a larger creation—the universe itself—and is thus subject to the same laws that govern the stars, the soil, and the sea.

Harmony and health, within the body and within the universe, depend on the careful balance of two opposing forces of nature called *yin* and *yang*. Furthermore, an energy called *qi* (pronounced "chee") permeates the entire universe and is the source of life and strength for all living matter. In Chinese medicine, all health care is designed to balance qi, to bring harmony between yin and yang. A primary method of releasing blocked qi is acupuncture: the use of needles to direct qi to organs or functions of the body or to disperse qi where it is excessive. As we'll discuss in Chapter 9, acupuncturists also use herbal medicine, massage, and a form of exercise known as *qi-gong*.

Aromatherapy. Essential oils that exude fragrances have been used as a component of medical treatment for centuries. Derived from plants, each fragrance has its own distinct odor which stimulates an array of emotional and psychological responses, which in turn cause certain physical reactions to occur that can help to heal the body.

Aromatherapists maintain that each plant has its own set of specific characteristics, based upon where it was grown and under what conditions. Pine trees, for instance, are able to grow and flourish even in the coldest winters and hottest summers and thus represent stability and fortitude. Aromatherapists believe that the scent of pine will stimulate a similar mood or response in anyone who is exposed to it. Chapter 8 discusses the oils that aromatherapists would use to treat someone with heart disease, such as arnica, which stimulates circulation, and lavender, which promotes a state of relaxation.

Ayurveda. Developed in India in about the fifth century B.C., Ayurveda, like Chinese medicine, considers a person's health within a cosmic context. Within the human body, universal force exists as an energy or life force called prana. Prana provides every human being the vitality and endurance to live in harmony with the universe, as well as offers the body the power to heal itself. Through examination of the tongue, pulse, facial features, and history, the Ayurvedic practitioner looks for imbalances which will lead to impurities blocking the circulatory system and causing heart disease. Treatment can include diet, yoga, herbs, breathing and meditation exercises.

Chiropractic. According to the theory behind chiropractic therapy, the spine is the wellspring from which the body's "innate intelligence" is derived. If the vertebrae of the spine are not properly aligned, the nerve impulses stemming from the spine cannot flow freely to distribute this innate intelligence to other parts of the body. Disease or ill health is the result. Chiropractors working with people who have heart disease concentrate on releasing the spinal nerves that affect the heart. As you'll discover in Chapter 11, in addition to massaging and manipulating the spine, many chiropractors also offer dietary advice and recommend exercises to promote blood flow to the heart and spine.

Herbal medicine. Essentially, herbal medicine is based on a holistic approach to health. It uses plant substances to stimulate the body to return to that state of internal balance we call health and to aid in natural healing. Though herbs are medicines, they are much safer than chemical drugs because they are less potent, more recognizable to the body as natural substances, and usually used in combinations that minimize side effects.

Like most other systems of natural health, herbal therapy is highly individualized. Herbal prescriptions are not based on a diagnosis of a specific disease, necessarily, but rather on the needs of each person based on his or her symptoms. In other words, an herbalist will treat you for high blood pressure or atherosclerosis in an entirely different way from another person with the same medical diagnosis but a different physiology and emotional makeup.

By careful questioning, the herbalist finds the causes of illness and prescribes treatment tailored to that individual's requirements. In addition to preparing herbal treatments, herbalists help people recognize and accept their own responsibility for their health and well-being. Advice on nutrition, exercise, and other lifestyle habits that affect the body's ability to remain in balance is thus also given. Therapy is not meant to merely provide relief, but to create long-lasting benefits by restoring the body to its natural state of health. How herbal therapy is used to treat heart disease is discussed in Chapter 12.

Homeopathy. Homeopathy is another system of medicine that attempts to harness the body's own healing power to fight disease and to maintain health. Developed in the early nineteenth century by German doctor Samuel Hahnemann, homeopathy is based on the principle that "like cures like." This theory postulates that medications should be given not to counteract the symptoms of illness, as they are in mainstream medicine. Instead, homeopathy uses highly diluted substances (called remedies) which would cause symptoms in full doses but in their diluted form stimulate a response in the body to bring it back into balance.

Like the above systems, homeopathy would not look at heart disease alone, but would look exhaustively at all your symptoms. The homeopath even wants to know such details as what hour your symptoms worsen or what side you like to sleep on, in order to settle on the ideal remedy.

Now that you've gained an understanding of natural medicine in general, it's time to learn a little about heart disease itself. Chapter 2 will provide you with some general information. Then, Chapter 3 will help answer any additional questions you might have about choosing an alternative therapy to treat your particular condition.

"The enlightened

heart is

its own heaven;

the ignorant

heart is

its own hell."

Doolittle,
Chinese Vocabulary
1872

Understanding Your Cardiovascular System

2

No organ of the body carries as much emotional and psychological weight as the human heart. We think of it not only as a pump that delivers blood through the body, but as a reservoir of emotion, morality, and thought. In every world society, from the ashrams of India to the operating rooms of modern American hospitals, the heart holds deep cultural and philosophical meaning. Indeed, only the coldest, most methodical cardiologist views this organ as a mere mechanical device.

Today, in the United States and in much of the industrialized world, the heart is in trouble. The whole circulatory system, in fact, is adversely affected by our modern American lifestyle. The food we eat, the exercise we fail to obtain, and the stress we feel are undermining the heart's ability to transport oxygen and nutrients through the bloodstream.

According to the latest statistics released by the National High Blood Pressure Education Program in October, 1994, an estimated 50 million Americans have high blood pressure and about 35 million have some degree of heart disease. Every year, these conditions result in approximately 1.5 million heart attacks and 500,000 strokes. More than 800,000 of these heart attacks and strokes are fatal. In addition to costing almost a million lives each year, cardiovascular disease exacts an enormous financial penalty as well: The American Heart Association estimates that Americans spend approximately $120 billion to treat cardiovascular disease every year.

The enormous burden cardiovascular disease places on our health care system is due, in large part, to the tremendous technological advances that have been made in the practice of modern medicine. Diagnostic equipment is more sophisticated, surgical techniques more advanced, and drug therapy considerably more widespread. And, it must be stated, not all of the money spent on these advances has been wasted: Without question, modern medicine has helped save lives that might have been lost to heart attack, stroke, or other complications of cardiovascular disease.

Fortunately, however, the limits of technology are being recognized by mainstream physicians as well as average American citizens. Slowly but surely, we are beginning to see that maintaining health and preventing disease should be our true goals and that technology cannot master these things for us. Only by taking control of our own bodies and spirits will the tide of cardiovascular disease be turned.

The good news is that this message has already reached many people: Physicians estimate that in the past twenty years about 10 million fewer Americans have developed high blood pressure, and some 200,000 strokes and an even greater number of heart attacks have been prevented. Most of this decline in cardiovascular disease may be due to drug therapy and surgery, but some is due to a fundamental change in the way we live. Fewer Americans smoke cigarettes or consume toxic quantities of fat, and more of us are realizing the benefits of exercise and peace of mind.

Chances are you or someone close to you has heart disease, high blood pressure, or another form of cardiovascular disease. You are searching for more natural and fundamental ways to restore your health and prevent further damage from being done. Before we discuss the many alternative treatments available to you, it is important that you learn about the cardiovascular system—how it works and what can go wrong.

Your Cardiovascular System at Work

Your cardiovascular system is made up of a vast network of blood vessels with a hollow muscular pump, the heart, at its center. The heart and blood vessels work together to deliver oxygen and nutrients to body organs and to remove waste products from tissue cells.

HEART FACTS

Your Hardest Working Muscle

- Each beat of the heart transports oxygen and nutrients to nourish 300 trillion cells.

- In one year, the human heart beats 3 million times.

- During exercise or stress, the heart may pump ten times as much blood as it does at rest.

- The heart beats approximately once a second and sends about 5 quarts of blood coursing through the circulatory system every minute.

- In total area, the capillary walls are equal to about 60,000 to 70,000 square feet, or roughly the area of one and a half football fields.

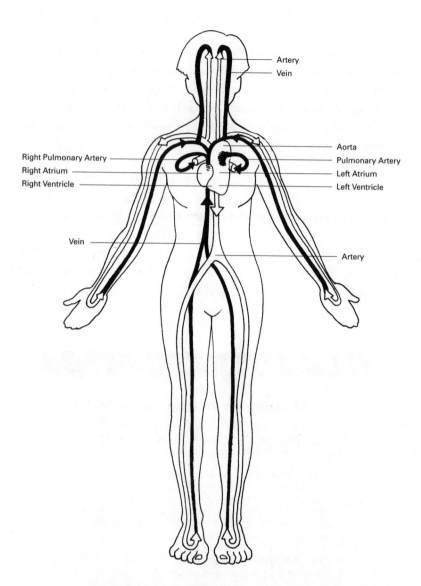

Artery
Vein

Aorta
Pulmonary Artery
Left Atrium
Left Ventricle

Right Pulmonary Artery
Right Atrium
Right Ventricle

Vein

Artery

The vascular system sends blood around the body in a continuous circuit, the arteries delivering oxygen and nutrients from the heart to body organs and tissues and the veins returning deoxygenated blood back to the heart and waste products to the liver and kidneys for removal. At the center of this cycle is the heart, the hardest working organ of the body.

The heart first sends blood to the lungs to pick up oxygen. It then pumps the oxygenated blood to the rest of the body and back through a system of tubes known as the vascular system. Stretched end to end, the blood vessels of your vascular system measure about 60,000 miles, but it takes just one minute for blood to complete one full circuit of the cardiovascular system.

To say that the human body works like an efficient machine is to make a vast understatement. Using a highly complex internal communications network that puts AT&T to shame, our various organ systems usually work together in the perfect harmony we know as health. Perhaps most amazing of all is that the majority of these functions are performed silently, unconsciously. We are usually quite oblivious to our inner workings: We read books, play tennis, digest food, and make love completely unaware of the number of hormones, enzymes, muscles, and nerves required to keep us on the go. Our hearts beat, steadily and almost silently, sending through a series of blood vessels the nutrients our body needs to perform its ordinary, everyday miracles.

When all goes well, the heart and blood vessels work in remarkable coordination to provide our bodies with all the nutrients we require to survive and thrive. However, there are several common ailments that may affect the cardiovascular system and thus the health of the entire body. These conditions, which include hypertension (high blood pressure), atherosclerosis (often caused by an excess of cholesterol), and heart disease, will be described in more detail later in this chapter. For now, it is important for you to determine if you or someone close to you is at risk of developing a disease that will adversely affect the health of the heart and blood vessels.

Determining Your Risk

Are you at risk of developing heart disease? If you are at risk, is there anything you can do to prevent it? If you already have heart

---

Risk Factors for Cardiovascular Disease

Risk factors are behaviors or conditions
that contribute to disease.
How many of these apply to you?

UNCONTROLLABLE	CONTROLLABLE
Heredity	Cigarette smoking
Age	Obesity
Race	Lack of exercise
Gender	Stress
	Diet (high-salt, high-cholesterol)

---

disease, high blood pressure, or high cholesterol levels, is there anything you can do to keep these conditions from causing a heart attack or stroke? The good news is that, in most cases, *cardiovascular disease may be preventable*—if you know its risk factors and how they may apply to you.

Risk factors are those conditions and/or habits associated with the increased likelihood of developing a disease. Cigarette smoking, for instance, is a risk factor for the development of heart disease and of lung cancer because chemicals in the smoke damage the arteries and lung tissue. High blood pressure itself is a risk factor for other cardiovascular diseases, including stroke and coronary heart disease.

The likelihood that you, as an individual, will develop a certain disease is influenced by both uncontrollable and controllable risk factors. If someone with sickle-cell anemia, for instance, inherited the disorder from his or her parents, the genetic factor that caused the disease is uncontrollable.

Other risk factors, however, are controllable. If you stop smoking, for instance, you've eliminated that particular risk factor for heart disease (as well as for a host of other lethal conditions, including lung cancer and high blood pressure). The following quiz can help you assess your risk.

Your Cardiovascular Self-Test

How old are you?
Under 40 (score 1 point)
40-55 (score 2 points)
Over 60 (score 3 points) _____

Have any of your close relatives—mother, father, sister, brother, aunt, uncle—had a stroke or heart attack?
No (1 point)
Yes, one relative (2 points)
Yes, more than one relative (3 points) _____

How often do you consume red meat and/or cheese?
Twice a week or less (1 point)
Three times a week (2 points)
More than three times a week (3 points) _____

How often do you eat fried foods?
Twice a week or less (1 point)
Three times a week (2 points)
More than three times a week (3 points) _____

How often do you consume fresh fruit and vegetables?
Three times each day (1 point)
Once a day (2 points)
Less than five times per week (3 points) _____

Do you smoke?
> I have never smoked/I gave up smoking
> > five years ago or more (1 point)
> I gave up smoking less than five years ago (2 points)
> I smoke 10 or more cigarettes a day (3 points) _____

Do you exercise on a regular basis?
> I participate in vigorous exercise (running, cycling,
> > swimming, etc.) at least three times a week (1 point)
> I am active once or twice a week (2 points)
> I lead a sedentary life (3 points) _____

Are you overweight?
> I am of normal weight or less than 10 pounds
> > overweight (1 point)
> I am between 10 and 20 pounds overweight (2 points)
> I am more than 20 pounds overweight (3 points) _____

Do you have a history of diabetes?
> No (1 point)
> Yes (3 points) _____

Do you regularly add salt to food while cooking?
> No (1 point)
> Yes (3 points) _____

How often do you eat processed foods or food from a fast food restaurant?
> Less than three times a week (1 point)
> Three times a week (2 points)
> Every day (3 points) _____

How often and how much do you drink alcoholic beverages?
> One to two drinks per day (1 point)
> Never (2 points)
> More than two drinks per day (3 points) _____

How do you react to stress?

I feel a sense of purpose when faced with a
professional or personal challenge (1 point)
I feel that life is a constant struggle and sometimes
feel frustrated and angry (2 points)
I feel trapped in a hard, sad, endless struggle
against impossible odds (3 points) _____

How often do you meditate or practice another relaxation method?

Three or more times per week (1 point)
Once a week (2 points)
Never (3 points) _____

Your Total_____

Calculating and Evaluating Your Score

28–42: Cardiac Red Alert. Your score indicates that you
are at very high risk for heart disease and high blood
pressure. If you do not already know the status of
your cardiovascular health, see a physician immediately for an evaluation.

14–27: Warning. If you're not careful, the food you eat and
the lifestyle you lead may eventually cause your
blood pressure to become elevated and your arteries
to develop atherosclerosis.

13 or Below: Stay On Guard. So far, you've managed to
avoid many of the common pitfalls on the road to
cardiovascular health, but it's important to keep
yourself on track.

Keep in mind that risk factors for cardiovascular disease are cumulative—the more that apply to you, the more likely you are to have a damaged heart and vessels. In other words, someone who smokes, has diabetes, and is obese has a much greater chance of developing heart disease than a nonsmoking, nondiabetic person who needs to lose weight.

This test is not meant to frighten you unduly. Just because you have a moderate or even very high risk of cardiovascular disease does not mean that you will actually suffer from it. It simply indicates that you are *more likely* to develop high blood pressure and/or heart disease than someone with low risk. This book will show you ways to reduce your risks and help keep your cardiovascular system healthy.

What Can Go Wrong

Often when we focus on one specific disease, we tend to lose sight of this most important aspect of human physiology: No one system of the body is separate from the others. To understand cardiovascular disease, for instance, we must go far beyond the heart and vessels and explore the kidneys, the glands, and the nervous system.

In addition, as we'll explore more fully throughout the book, looking at the body itself, without taking into consideration the emotions and the intellect, is just as shortsighted as looking at the heart in isolation from the arteries or the kidneys. Nevertheless, it is important to understand, from a purely physiological perspective, the many different forms of cardiovascular disease and how they may affect your overall health.

ATHEROSCLEROSIS: CLOGGED VESSELS

The overwhelming majority of diseases of the heart muscle (myocardium) are caused by atherosclerosis, or hardening of the arteries. This is the name given to the buildup of plaque—made up of fatty substances and blood clots—on the inner walls of the arteries. This buildup is a gradual process, one that may take decades before any symptoms of cardiovascular damage (known as atherosclerotic cardiovascular disease or ASCVD) appear.

HEART FACTS

Heart Disease— Not for Men Only

- Heart attacks are the leading killer of women, claiming six times the number of lives lost to breast cancer.

- Of the 500,000 fatal heart attacks in the United States every year, 247,000 occur in women.

- Women who have a heart attack are twice as likely as men to die within the following few weeks.

- Age is a major risk factor for women: Of the 247,000 fatal heart attacks every year, only about 6,500 occur in women under the age of 65. Estrogen, a female hormone, is believed to protect the heart and blood vessels from the effects of atherosclerosis. Women are at higher risk after menopause, when the body produces little of the hormone.

- Medical researchers at the National Institutes of Health are launching a $500 million, 14-year study of 140,000 postmenopausal women called the Women's Health Initiative. Research will explore the effects of the diet, smoking, and other factors on women's risk of developing cardiovascular disease and other common health problems, including osteoporosis and breast cancer.

The plaque gathers in response to damage to the inner wall of an artery. This damage can come from many sources, and this is where lifestyle decisions have a big effect. Fatty and fried foods promote arterial damage and plaque buildup. High blood pressure pushes against arterial walls with a greater than normal force and thus damages the lining. Toxic substances such as nicotine and cocaine irritate and damage the arterial lining. And hormones secreted during periods of high stress have an abrasive effect as well.

Whatever the initial injury, the body has special cells that act to heal the damaged places by sticking to the area in question. These special cells are fats, including cholesterol, and over time they accumulate at the site of the damage, further blocking the artery. If plaque builds up in the coronary arteries, it can cause coronary heart disease. If it's building up in the cerebral arteries, it can cause a stroke. And if it builds up in the arteries of the legs, claudication (lack of blood supply) to the legs can occur.

Coronary heart disease is a term used to describe several different disorders of the heart muscle that are caused by restriction or blockage of its blood supply. The disorders range from the warning pain called angina to the injury and even death of parts of the heart muscle caused by a heart attack.

Many people experience pain called *angina pectoris* as their heart muscle becomes deprived of oxygen. Angina usually occurs when the heart's workload increases and the heart cannot get enough oxygen to enable it to perform, such as during or after exercise or some other strenuous physical activity or when a person is experiencing strong emotion (like anger).

The pain of angina is usually located in the center of the chest, but may radiate to or occur only in the neck, shoulder, arm, or lower jaw. No permanent damage to the heart occurs during an angina attack, but it is a warning sign that your cardiovascular system may be in trouble.

Heart attack is the most serious consequence of coronary artery disease. A heart attack occurs when an area of the heart muscle is so severely deprived of blood that it can no longer survive. Heart attacks are also called *myocardial infarctions*. (*Myo* means "muscle," *cardio* means relating to the heart, and *infarct* is a word used to describe the area of dead tissue.)

Most heart attacks occur when a coronary artery already narrowed by atherosclerosis is suddenly and completely blocked by a blood clot or muscular spasm. When such a sudden blockage occurs, blood flow to the heart is immediately cut off, causing the death of the heart tissue nourished by the affected artery.

HIGH BLOOD PRESSURE: THE SILENT KILLER

With each heartbeat, 2 to 3 ounces of freshly oxygenated blood are forced out of the heart and into general circulation. To keep the blood flowing through the 60,000 miles of vessels, a certain amount of force is required. This force is called *blood pressure*. At the head of the blood pressure system is the heart, but the arterioles, the smallest arteries, also play a large role in determining the amount of pressure in the vessels throughout the body. To raise blood pressure, the arterioles narrow; to lower it, they open up. While the force required to keep blood moving through the body originates in the heart and vessels, three other body systems work together to control the blood pressure: the kidneys (which help to regulate the amount of fluid circulating in the body), the nervous system (which helps control the contraction and dilation of the blood vessels), and the endocrine system (which produces hormones that tell the other systems what to do).

About 90 to 95 percent of all cases of high blood pressure (or hypertension) are classified as *essential hypertension*, which means that doctors can't determine a precise cause for it. Because the blood pressure system is so complicated and involves so many different components, it's often difficult to pinpoint exactly what's causing high blood pressure in a given individual. In about 10 percent of cases, there's an underlying or secondary cause. Kidney disease could be the culprit or it may be due to an external factor, such as the side effects of certain prescription drugs.

STROKE: BRAIN ATTACK

A stroke often occurs when the brain is deprived of its blood supply by the same process that causes a heart attack—namely atherosclerosis. Although stroke affects the brain, it is not technically a neurological disease. Instead, it is a disease of the blood vessels that feed the brain.

Just as high blood pressure is called "the silent killer" because of its lack of overt symptoms, strokes can also occur without warning. However, about 10 percent of all people who have a stroke are warned in advance that all is not well. They experience a TIA (transient ischemic attack), often called a "mini-stroke," which involves a temporary loss of blood to an area of the brain. A TIA resolves itself within 24 hours or so. Once a TIA has occurred, it tends to recur, or lead to strokes, unless the underlying cause is eliminated.

OTHER CARDIAC CONDITIONS

In addition to high blood pressure and coronary artery disease, there are several common conditions that can affect the heart and circulatory system. Some of them are congenital (present at birth) and others develop at a later date. The most common are arrhythmias and mitral valve prolapse.

Arrhythmias (also known as dysrhythmias) are abnormalities in the electrical current that stimulates the heart muscle. These abnormalities produce irregular heartbeats. Most irregular heartbeats are harmless, except when other heart problems are also present. An arrhythmia is not necessarily an indication of heart disease, but some types of arrhythmia are potentially fatal. For that reason you should see your doctor about any heartbeat irregularity.

Mitral valve prolapse is an abnormality in which the flaps of tissue that make up this heart valve are larger than normal. This defect causes the valve to close improperly and, often, allows blood to leak backward. The vast majority of individuals with this condition suffer no symptoms and are not in any danger from it. However, its symptoms, when they do occur, often mimic those of angina, including chest pain, dizziness, and palpitations.

Diagnosing Heart Disease

Cardiovascular disease can sneak up on you. You might not be aware that you are ill before significant damage has already been done. That's why it is important for you to visit a doctor—mainstream or alternative—to monitor the health of your heart and blood vessels. *Diagnosis is* not *the same thing as treatment.* If you regularly visit a holistic practitioner, it is likely that he or she will suggest that you see a mainstream physician to evaluate your condition if heart disease is suspected.

It is important that you take advantage of all available techniques for diagnosing cardiovascular disease. Once your condition is known, you can then make an informed decision on which of the many mainstream and alternative treatment options are best for you. In other words, the results of the tests and procedures performed by a mainstream physician will be very useful to an alternative practitioner in determining appropriate therapy. In Chapter 1, we explored all of the therapies available to you, both mainstream and alternative.

When you visit a mainstream physician, the first thing he or she will do is take a complete medical history. When taking a history, your doctor will want to know about any medication you are on. He or she will want to know whether you or any other members of your family have ever been diagnosed with high blood pressure, heart disease, kidney disease, diabetes, or have experienced symptoms of stroke. In other words, the doctor will ask you many of the same questions asked in the "Cardiovascular Self-Test" earlier in this chapter, which is why it might be helpful for you to complete the test before visiting a physician.

Next, your physician will perform a physical exam. The order in which your doctor decides to perform the physical exam is arbitrary, but for simplicity's sake, we'll start from the head and work our way down. Your doctor will first look into your eyes with an instrument called an ophthalmoscope, which shines a very bright light onto your retina (the light-sensitive area at the back of your eye). The blood vessels here are easily visible, and your doctor will be able to tell if high blood pressure and/or atherosclerosis has damaged them. He or she will probably feel your neck for an enlarged thyroid gland—since an overactive thyroid gland can occasionally cause high blood pressure and an underactive thyroid can raise lipid levels—and will check the arteries in your neck.

The doctor will feel manually for your heartbeat, listen to your heart rhythms with a stethoscope, and check your lungs for signs of fluid not being pumped adequately by the heart. He or she will examine your abdomen, checking for abnormalities in your kidneys, and will take the pulses in your arms and legs. In this way, your doctor will be able to assess the condition of your blood vessels throughout your body.

In addition to the physical exam, you'll have tests to measure your blood pressure and to determine the health of your blood. These tests are standard procedures usually performed in your doctor's office during a regular physical checkup.

MEASURING BLOOD PRESSURE

A blood pressure measurement consists of two numbers separated by a slashmark. The upper number, called *systolic pressure*, is a measurement of pressure in the artery when the heart has pumped blood into it during its contraction (called the systole). The lower number, called *diastolic pressure*, is a measurement of how much pressure remains in the artery during the heart's relaxation (called the diastole).

A blood pressure exam is relatively simple and completely painless. Blood pressure is measured with an instrument called a sphygmomanometer, which allows physicians to calculate how hard the heart is pumping and how much the blood vessels must contract to push the blood along. The sphygmomanometer is made up of three components: an inflatable rubber cuff attached to a gauge that resembles a thermometer, and a stethoscope. The cuff is wrapped snugly around your arm, air is pumped into it until the cuff is tight enough to keep blood from flowing, then released. Your doctor listens through the stethoscope for the sound of the first spurt of blood as it passes through the artery, this is the systolic pressure. When the doctor no long hears any sounds through the stethoscope, the diastolic pressure is read. Your blood pressure is determined by these two numbers.

How high is too high? Although general categories have been established, the truth is that no exact dividing line exists between normal and high blood pressure. The National High Blood Pressure Education Program recently revised its classification of blood pressure into approximately five separate categories. Anything reading between 110/70 and 140/90 is within the normal range. High blood pressure is any reading higher than about 140 systolic and 90 diastolic.

It should be noted that blood pressure is a highly individual matter. Your own "perfect" blood pressure is determined by your weight, height, age, and other individual physical characteristics factors. Generally speaking, however, the lower your blood pressure the better: Someone with a blood pressure of 110/70 runs fewer cardiovascular health risks than someone with a blood pressure of 120/80. In turn, the person with a 120/80 reading may fare better in the long run than the person whose pressure is measured at 135/85.

DETERMINING THE HEALTH OF YOUR BLOOD

Measuring the amount of fats or lipids circulating in your blood will help to determine your risk of atherosclerosis. Your blood lipid profile is determined by testing blood drawn from a vein in your arm. In an effort to standardize the results, many physicians now recommend that this blood test be performed after a 12-hour fast.

It should be noted that when we talk about "fat," we're usually discussing the larger category of body substances called lipids. Lipids include fats, fatty acids, sterols, and other compounds that circulate in our bloodstream and are part of our cells. Although not all lipids are fats, the two terms tend to be used interchangeably, which can be misleading. Cholesterol, for instance, is not a fat, but a fatlike lipid called a sterol.

Cholesterol is essential for a number of vital body processes, like nerve function and cell reproduction. The antistress hormones hydrocortisone and aldosterone, for example, and the sex hormones estrogen and testosterone are produced from cholesterol. Although your body can't survive without cholesterol, that doesn't mean you have to consume it. Your liver manufactures all it needs from other materials. The average American diet, however, includes 600 to 1,500 milligrams (mg) of cholesterol each day, far more than you or anyone else needs.

Your doctor will discuss with you the results of your blood lipid profile. However, the National Cholesterol Education Program, sponsored by the National Institutes of Health, recommends that total blood cholesterol should be below 200 milligrams/decaliters. A reading of between 200 and 239 is borderline, and any reading over 240 milligrams/decaliters is considered high. In Chapter 4, you'll learn the best ways to cut down on the amount of cholesterol you eat so that your heart and blood vessels have the best possible chance of remaining healthy and strong.

DETERMINING THE HEALTH OF YOUR HEART

As discussed above, your doctor will first listen to your heart through a stethoscope to check its size, the rate at which it beats, and the types of sounds it makes. If your doctor has any reason to suspect that your heart is diseased, you may need further tests. If you are a man over the age of 40, a woman past the age of menopause, or if you have one or more risk factors for heart disease, your physician may also decide to use one or more of the following procedures as a screening method to rule out heart disease. The results of these tests can serve as a baseline with which to compare the results of future tests.

Unless you have serious heart disease requiring surgery, none of the tests a mainstream doctor may recommend are dangerous or invasive. In fact, most of these tests are tests that any legitimate holistic practitioner would insist on having performed before any treatment is prescribed. The most common and relatively risk-free diagnostic procedures for heart disease include the electrocardiogram (ECG), the exercise stress test, and the echocardiogram.

Electrocardiogram. Also known as an ECG, this is a commonly done screening test, but not a very good indicator of coronary heart disease. An ECG gives a record of the heart's electrical patterns while at rest. In a healthy person, the passage of electrical impulses through the heart follows a regular sequence. If there is any abnormality, this pattern is altered. By observing the electrical patterns your heart produces, your doctor can identify areas of the heart muscle that may have been damaged by coronary heart disease, as well as detect thickening of heart muscle walls or irregular heartbeats (arrhythmias).

The electrocardiogram is performed by attaching electrodes to the chest, wrists, and ankles. In most cases, an ECG is performed while you are lying down. Although completely painless, some patients complain that the substance used to attach the electrodes causes temporary skin irritation.

Stress test. This examination is used to measure the electrical patterns of the heart during exertion. It is a very common and usually painless and risk-free procedure. You will probably be asked to walk or jog on a treadmill or ride a stationary bike and your heart will be monitored continuously by an ECG. The idea is to increase your heart's need for blood and oxygen by raising your heart rate slowly to a predetermined level. Such a test will reveal blockage to blood flow that is only evident when the heart is stressed as it exercises.

If the results of your stress test and/or ECG are abnormal, your doctor may recommend another type of stress test called a thallium scan. The thallium scan produces a visual, dynamic picture of the part of the heart muscle that is not receiving enough blood during exercise.

Echocardiogram. This painless procedure uses ultrasound (extremely high-frequency sound waves) to produce an image of the heart, and gives a clear picture of the heart's size, how it is actually functioning, and if there are any valve abnormalities or other structural changes. The test is performed by placing a transducer—a device that emits ultrasound waves—on your chest. The image produced by the sound waves bouncing off the heart is projected onto a monitor and recorded on videotape.

Coronary angiography. If your doctor suspects that heart disease has caused serious damage to your heart muscle, if you've suffered a heart attack, or if your physician thinks you may require heart surgery, another procedure may be performed. Called a *cardiac catheterization (arteriogram)*, this surgical procedure determines the degree and location of any blockage that may have been detected in earlier tests. It is performed by first giving local anesthesia in the right groin region, then inserting a tube into a large artery in the groin (the femoral artery), which leads directly to the heart. A dye is injected through the tube, and an x-ray called a coronary angiogram is taken. If coronary artery disease is present, the dye will not fill that area, and it will show up on the x-ray.

Although catheterization of the coronary arteries is quite useful in diagnosing heart disease, it is not without some risk. In rare cases, catheterization may cause blockage where the catheter is inserted, heart attack, or other serious complications. Please discuss the matter thoroughly with your physician and seek a second opinion if you have any questions about this procedure.

When it comes to your health, knowledge is power. In this chapter, you've learned how your heart and blood vessels work to nourish your body. In Chapter 3, we'll try to answer some of your questions about the many natural options available to help you keep your cardiovascular system healthy and/or to repair any damage to it that may have already occurred.

"There are only two ways to live. One is as though nothing is a miracle, the other as though everything is a miracle."

Albert Einstein

Choosing an Alternative

$\mathcal{I}$n early 1993, a landmark in Western medicine was reached when the National Institutes of Health (NIH) opened the doors of its Office of Alternative Medicine. That the NIH, long a bastion of mainstream medical research, would devote resources to exploring such alternatives as acupuncture, homeopathy, and meditation gratified the growing numbers of physicians and patients who had been using these therapies for many years.

The NIH's decision was no doubt influenced by reports that more and more Americans are using alternative medicine every day. Another citadel of mainstream medicine, the *New England Journal of Medicine,* reported in 1992 that an astounding one in three Americans had used some form of alternative therapy as part of their medical therapy in 1990, a number that will no doubt increase as the advantages of alternative care become more accepted by mainstream institutions like the NIH and better known to the public at large. In fact, today more than twenty medical schools offer courses on holistic and alternative medicine studies for their students, and the University of Arizona is now in the process of creating a residency program in "Integrated Medicine" which will blend standard and alternative approaches.

Among those who will benefit most from the increased understanding of the principles of alternative medicine are the millions of Americans who suffer from cardiovascular disease or who are at risk of developing it. In fact, when it comes to treating heart disease, the line between mainstream and alternative medicine is becoming quite blurry: Proper nutrition, exercise, and stress reduction—all fundamental principles of most alternative therapies—are now also recognized as essential components of any successful heart disease treatment plan.

More and more Americans are beginning to search for new answers to age-old questions about the true meaning of health: Instead of settling for patching up a damaged heart or taking pills to lower blood pressure, people are now willing to invest time and energy to creating a longer-lasting, more natural state of balance.

Choosing to treat cardiovascular disease without drugs or surgery involves making a larger commitment to your health than you may have made in the past. In addition, there are aspects of alternative health care that you may find unfamiliar and, at least at first, a little uncomfortable. Most forms of alternative therapy, for instance, require that you gain a more intimate knowledge of your body through exercise and massage. You may even have to get used to your practitioner examining your body in a different way than your mainstream physician has in the past.

In order to gain the most benefit from natural medicine, you'll also need to learn to truly relax your body and mind. For many people, this experience involves exploring emotional and spiritual issues that may have been ignored or suppressed for many years. Although exciting, and ultimately liberating, such work requires some extra motivation, strength, and guidance.

For the vast majority of people who choose to replace or supplement their mainstream health care with more natural approaches, the benefits they reap from their decision are well worth the physical and emotional effort. It is important, however, to gain some understanding of what various alternative therapies require of you before you become involved with them. The following quiz will help you sort out some of the questions you may have about alternative medicine and how it might fit into your life.

Your Alternative Medicine Quick Quiz

The questions in this quiz focus on four different issues you should consider when looking for an alternative approach to health and health care. The four questions in Part A concern the physical aspects of health care; Part B looks at diet and nutrition; Part C helps you focus on your emotional and spiritual side; and Part D examines practical matters such as finances and access to alternative health care facilities.

Answer yes or no to these sixteen questions then check with the answer guide that follows to find out what you should look for, or look to avoid, in choosing an alternative therapy.

Part A

1. I enjoy being massaged or touched by a qualified practitioner. _____

2. I am willing to experience some discomfort during my treatment. _____

3. I tolerate needles well. _____

4. I enjoy physical exercise or am willing to make exercise a part of my life. _____

Part B

1. I am willing to change my diet. _____
2. I am willing to learn about nutrition. _____
3. I prepare most of my meals at home. _____
4. I accept that vitamins and minerals are helpful in treating disease. _____

Part C

1. I accept that emotions play a role in health and healing. _____
2. I can accept scientifically unproven remedies. _____
3. I understand that restoring my body to health will take time and effort. _____
4. I now include meditation as part of my daily life or would like to in the future. _____

Part D

1. I have easy access to one or more alternative practitioners. _____
2. I have the time and the desire to make and keep appointments for alternative treatments. _____
3. I have some discretionary income to pay for alternative treatments. _____
4. I can accept alternative therapies that have not been proven scientifically. _____

THE ANSWER GUIDE

Take a look at your answers. Were most of them "yes"? Was there one category, or more, in which you answered several questions with a "no"? As you'll see in the following guide, your answers to these questions will help you find the type or types of natural therapy that best suit your own distinct personality and personal needs.

A: The physical. Many natural approaches to health care require patients to establish a new relationship with their own bodies and, in some cases, with their physicians or practitioners.

If you dislike being touched by your doctor, then therapies that use massage or other types of physical manipulation as part of their approach may not be for you. Unless you think you can learn to overcome this aversion, it might be best for you to avoid acupuncture, Ayurvedic medicine, and chiropractic, all of which use physical therapy to a large extent. Likewise, if you are afraid of needles, then acupuncture is not for you unless you can easily put aside your fears. Being tense and uncomfortable will work directly against the state of balance and relaxation that is the goal of natural medicine.

However, if one or more of these therapies interest you despite your fears or aversions, then you should consider discussing with a practitioner how the philosophy behind the treatment can be used to help you without using the elements that make you uncomfortable.

Whether you like it or not, however, physical activity of some kind will soon be a larger part of your life if you've been diagnosed with cardiovascular disease. Increased physical activity is a key element in the treatment of cardiovascular disease both from a mainstream and from an alternative perspective. Fortunately, as you'll discover in Chapter 6, exercise doesn't have to mean slogging away on a stationary bicycle or struggling to lift weights in a gym. Instead, you'll learn ways to get your heart pumping, your muscles working, and your spirit lifted by choosing a physical activity that you enjoy.

B: The nutritional. Along with adding exercise to your daily life, treating cardiovascular disease naturally will most likely require you to make significant changes to your diet. Indeed, there is no approach, mainstream or alternative, that ignores the impact of diet on the cardiovascular system. Reducing fats, adding fiber, and eliminating preservatives and other additives are just some of the dietary modifications you'll need to make in order to help your heart and blood vessels heal.

As anyone who's ever dieted can tell you, making such major changes in your day-to-day habits may seem difficult and daunting. The first step is to learn as much as possible about nutrition, both from a mainstream perspective and from within the context of the alternative method you choose to follow. Understanding why certain foods will help or harm you should make it easier for you to eat or avoid them. Some alternative therapies require stricter changes than others: Ayurvedic medicine, for instance, involves detoxifying the body with the use of certain herbs and a period of fasting, and, depending on your body type, the elimination of certain foods from the diet. If you eat most of your meals outside the home, or otherwise have little control over your daily menu, such a strategy may be difficult for you to follow.

Another important element in the treatment of heart disease through nutrition is the use of vitamin and mineral supplements. Recent studies have shown that certain substances, called antioxidants, may dramatically reduce the risk of cardiovascular disease. Since it may be difficult to obtain sufficient levels of antioxidants and other beneficial nutrients from our diets, many practitioners, both mainstream and alternative, are now suggesting that their patients take dietary supplements. If you feel uncomfortable taking pills, such an approach may not be for you, and you may have to work especially hard to get the nutrients you need from your diet.

As you'll see in Chapter 4, however, you should not feel overwhelmed at the prospect of starting "a diet." Such changes can be made relatively slowly, over time, until they become natural, enjoyable habits. Working carefully with your alternative practitioner and/or a nutritional therapist, you'll be able to design an appropriate eating plan for a healthy heart that does not unduly disrupt your life or render it devoid of culinary pleasure.

C: The emotional. Perhaps the most essential difference between mainstream and alternative medicine is the way in which the emotional and spiritual side of life is considered. Unlike mainstream medicine, most forms of natural therapy regard how you feel about your life as being just as important as how much cholesterol is circulating in your blood. In fact, the level of stress in one's life may directly impact the amount of cholesterol circulating in the blood: Without addressing the emotions, then, one aspect of the underlying physical problem is ignored altogether.

Such an approach to cardiovascular health, however, requires people to invest time and energy in an area of their lives they may have neglected in the past. If you're used to feeling better immediately because you've taken a pill or other prescription, looking at health in this way may seem time-consuming and ineffective—at least in the short term. Indeed, as discussed in Chapter 1, there are no quick fixes in alternative medicine. Patience is an essential part of the natural healing process.

Because emotional balance is an essential goal of natural medicine, learning to reduce the amount of stress in your life, as well as learning to better cope with the stress that remains, is an integral component of any natural treatment of cardiovascular disease. Meditation, biofeedback, and visualization are all methods of achieving emotional balance, and it is important that you remain open to exploring these methods as you strive toward health.

D: The practical. Quite apart from the personal factors that may lead you toward a particular form of health care, there are practical matters to consider as well. First and foremost is how much access you have to alternative medicine resources. If you have to drive several hours to visit a homeopath or acupuncturist, treatment for a chronic condition like heart disease with these methods may not be workable.

Time is another important consideration: Many alternative therapies require more frequent visits to a practitioner than you may be used to, especially at the beginning of a treatment plan. If you are often out of town or have other time constraints, you may want to steer away from those approaches. Acupuncture and chiropractic are particularly time-consuming, as they usually necessitate a continued course of therapy.

Another obstacle for many people is money. Although in the long term, alternative approaches to health care appear to be less expensive than mainstream technology and pharmacology, there may be an immediate impact on the pocketbook, primarily because most forms of health insurance do not yet cover alternative medicine.

Finally, one practical matter for you to consider is your own commitment to the process of natural healing. Many alternative therapies, despite having been practiced in other cultures for centuries, have not been proven according to Western medical standards. (Even many

Western drugs have not really been "proven" according to these ideal standards; anyone who takes an aspirin for a headache can attest to that.) If you are someone who needs to understand the scientific basis for a therapy before beginning it, many of these alternatives may be too challenging for you at this time. Homeopathy, for instance, is based on an understanding very different from that of the standard medical model. To attempt to work with a homeopath in treating your heart disease, therefore, requires that you accept the results without fully understanding the process.

As you can see, choosing the type of alternative medicine that is best for you may involve thinking about your life, your body, and your spirit in new ways. Because natural remedies, by their very nature, are safe and relatively free of side effects, you should feel a certain freedom to experiment with different therapies before choosing one over another.

In addition, you may decide to mix and match one or more types of approaches instead of using just one alternative method. Fortunately, many holistic practitioners either have more than one specialty or are involved in group practices. For example, an herbal medicine specialist may also be trained in aromatherapy or may share an office with an aromatherapist. If a person so chooses, both herbs and essential oils can be used as treatment.

No matter what type or types of natural therapy you choose, however, it is essential that you find qualified professionals to treat you. The following section offers a step-by-step guide to locating a reputable practitioner and establishing an effective, supportive relationship with him or her.

Becoming a Wise Alternative Health Care Consumer

Successful treatment of cardiovascular disease, whether by alternative or mainstream means, requires a partnership between you and the people who treat you, one that is built on mutual trust and respect.

You must feel confident in the practitioners' ability to help treat your health problems, and they must know vital, accurate information about your medical status and lifestyle in order to provide you with that help. Here are some guidelines that will help you accomplish these goals:

Obtain an accurate diagnosis. Before you decide upon an alternative therapy or practitioner, it is important for you to have certain tests and procedures performed. These tests are best done by a cardiologist at a hospital or clinic. Bring the results of these tests with you to your first appointment with an alternative practitioner.

Learn as much as possible about the alternative therapy or therapies that appeal to you. Knowledge is power, especially when it comes to health care. Read articles and books about the type of alternative care that appeals to you, talk to friends and acquaintances who use that method, and ask your mainstream physician for his or her opinion.

Check credentials carefully. To date, there are no national licensing requirements for most alternative medicine practitioners as there are for mainstream physicians. Instead, certification and licensing are done on a state-by-state basis. Ask your local department of health for the licensing requirements, certification, degrees, and diplomas you should look for in a holistic practitioner. To find out more information about a specific treatment or a specific practitioner, you may call a national association in the specialty field you are considering. (See *An Alternative Medicine Resource Guide*, p. 196)

Interview your prospective practitioner. It is often a good idea to make a short appointment with a practitioner, even before you decide to be examined by him or her. During this visit, you should take note of the office itself: Is it clean? Are you comfortable there? What are the billing procedures and are they willing to set up a payment plan for you? Is the staff friendly and accommodating? Do patient boundaries and confidentiality seem to be respected? When you meet with the practitioner, ask about how much experience he or she has had in treating cardiovascular disease. Find out how accessible he or she is between appointments and in case of emergencies. Although it is doubtful that you will feel completely comfortable with the practitioner during this first short meeting, it may be clear to you whether there is a potential for a close relationship. Trust your instincts. If you feel uneasy for any reason, you should not feel obligated to continue meeting with that practitioner.

Prepare for a long first appointment. Depending on the type of alternative therapy you've chosen to explore, your first appointment (other than the prospective interview) with a practitioner may last from 45 to 90 minutes. You'll probably find that most of that time is spent discussing matters you've never discussed with a physician before. You'll probably be asked detailed questions about your diet, your medical history, your exercise habits, and your feelings about the work you do and your personal life. Such information is crucial in developing a treatment plan for you, as a unique individual whose spirit and mind are as integral to health as is your body.

At the same time, you should feel comfortable asking your own questions about your condition, about the procedures your practitioner performs, and even about the questions he or she is asking you. Your practitioner should answer these questions in an open and honest way. If you feel you are not being listened to or respected, you have reason to look for another person to treat you.

Get a clear idea of what the suggested course of treatment involves. Discuss what to expect from a treatment *before* you agree to it. Ask the practitioner about what side effects or adverse reactions are possible from the suggested therapy. Find out how many appointments and how much time it will take before you see symptoms alleviated and improvement made in the health of your heart and blood vessels. Ask how much the treatment will cost. Although the course of treatment may change as therapy continues, a qualified practitioner should be able to give you a reasonable prognosis and timetable.

Establish a relationship between your mainstream and alternative practitioners. Ask your mainstream doctor if he or she would be willing to collaborate with an alternative practitioner on your care—and ask the same thing of any natural therapist you choose. With serious, chronic illnesses like heart disease, it is sensible to work toward having the best of both worlds: the lifesaving technology of Western medicine in cases of emergency and the natural, mind-body methods of healing implicit in alternative medicine. In Chapter 14, you'll see how mainstream and alternative medicine can work together to bring you closer to cardiovascular health.

Feel free to obtain a second opinion. If you feel uncertain about the approach your mainstream and/or alternative practitioner has chosen to treat your cardiovascular disease, you should find another qualified doctor or practitioner to evaluate your case.

Don't be afraid to experiment. What works for one individual may not work for another, and that is especially true when it comes to health care. If the type of therapy you've chosen, through your own research or with advice from a friend, does not suit you, you should feel free to explore another until you find one or a combination of approaches that is effective, safe, and comfortable.

Don't be afraid to change physicians or practitioners. If for any reason you are not happy with your current physician or alternative therapist, you should feel free to choose another. Such a decision should not be made lightly, especially if you've been under someone's care for some time. On the other hand, only by working within an atmosphere of mutual trust and respect will treatment for a chronic condition like heart disease work over the long term. Qualified practitioners should understand if you decide to leave them and should cooperate fully in providing your new physician with your records and other information.

Now that you've received a primer of sorts on the basics of alternative medicine, it's time to explore the various types of natural therapies used to treat cardiovascular disease. The next few chapters provide the fundamentals of any successful treatment plan: diet, exercise, and relaxation. Following those first-tier strategies are chapters covering other types of alternative care that may also help you on your journey toward true, long-lasting health. Read them carefully, and feel free to ask your mainstream or alternative practitioner any questions about how these treatments may apply to your specific cardiovascular problem.

"Thy food

be thy remedy."

Hippocrates

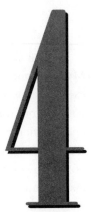

Eating Right for
a Healthy Heart

ake this short quiz to test your knowledge of nutrition and its relationship to heart disease. Mark each statement true or false.

_____ Cholesterol causes heart disease.
_____ All fat is bad.
_____ Carbohydrates make you fat.
_____ Extra protein makes you strong.
_____ Alcohol is always harmful.
_____ Counting calories is the only effective way to lose weight.

Give yourself 5 points for every statement you thought was true. The higher your score, the more you will gain from reading this chapter about nutrition—*because all of these statements are false.*

If you scored on the high side on this quiz, you're not alone. Myths about nutrition abound, and every day a new dietary theory explodes onto the front page of our newspapers. This chapter will help you sort out the myths from the facts. It will help you develop a balanced eating plan, one that will help return your cardiovascular system to a state of health in the most natural way possible. (It should be noted, however, that the information in this chapter is based on fairly mainstream concepts of nutrition. Many alternative therapies, particularly Ayurvedic and homeopathic medicine, may require that you follow very specific nutritional guidelines. Those guidelines will be covered in relevant chapters.)

Food and Cardiovascular Disease

To understand the relationship between cardiovascular disease and what you eat, we must turn our attention to atherosclerosis. Atherosclerosis occurs when the inner layer of the arteries becomes thickened, thus reducing the amount of blood that can flow through. When blood flow is restricted, cells do not receive the oxygen and other nutrients they need to survive, nor can they release waste materials into the bloodstream for elimination.

Atherosclerosis is a complicated process that usually takes place over a period of several decades. Exactly why it develops is still not completely understood. The most widely accepted theory proposes that atherosclerosis begins when a portion of a blood vessel is damaged.

No matter what the initial cause, an injury to a blood vessel triggers a response from the immune system: Specialized blood cells responsible for healing are attracted to the damaged area, as is collagen, a protein of the connective tissue. Platelets traveling in the bloodstream stick to the area as well. These substances adhere to the vessel, creating scar tissue over the injury. Over time, lipids as well as deposits of calcium may also accumulate at the site of the damage, further blocking the artery. Should atherosclerosis occur in a heart vessel or a vessel in the brain, or should a piece of plaque from another site break off and clog an artery in the heart or brain, a heart attack or stroke is the result.

Scientists have discovered many important links between what we eat and the process of atherosclerosis. First, certain nutritive substances, like magnesium, chromium, vitamin B_6, and niacin, lower the amount of fat in the blood. Other nutritive substances, like vitamins C, E, and A, and minerals like selenium and zinc, prevent fats from being able to damage blood vessels. (Some of these substances are called antioxidants; they'll be discussed later in the chapter and in Chapter 5.)

Second, what we eat may directly impact on the development of high blood pressure, a leading cause of initial damage to blood vessels. Eating too much sodium, eating too little potassium or magnesium, and drinking too much alcohol are a few of the ways that our diets may upset the delicate internal balance of blood pressure and thus lead to atherosclerosis.

Third, fats and fatlike materials called lipids and sterols are among the substances that attach to injured blood vessels. The most well known of these substances is cholesterol. Although the metabolism of cholesterol is extremely complex, it appears that the higher the level of cholesterol and fat in the bloodstream, the more likely atherosclerotic plaque is to form.

However, the level of cholesterol in the bloodstream and its ability to cause damage depend on a variety of factors, among them the amount of fat, antioxidants, and other substances, both beneficial and harmful, also present. Another element important in any discussion of cholesterol is the amount of sugar and simple carbohydrates (like refined white flour) consumed. These substances act on the body in two ways: First, they are more easily stored as fat than complex carbohydrates (like whole-wheat flour) or protein. Second, simple carbohydrates tend to raise the level of insulin in the body. Insulin is a hormone produced by the pancreas that allows blood sugar (called glucose) to leave the bloodstream and enter the cells to be used as energy. High levels of circulating glucose and insulin are linked to increased amounts of cholesterol in the blood as well as increased "stickiness" of platelets, both of which promote the development of atherosclerosis.

As you can see, your diet plays a large role in cardiovascular disease. In fact, through research performed by Dean Ornish, M.D., of the University of California and others, it has been found that the most effective—and completely natural—treatment of cardiovascular disease over the long term is dietary: If you eat enough of the right kinds of food, and limit your intake of substances known to be harmful, you can significantly reverse the damage that's already been done to your cardiovascular system and/or decrease your risk of developing cardiovascular disease in the future.

Learning about nutrition is important for everyone. Poor dietary habits, such as eating too much fat and not enough fiber, are related to several serious health problems, including certain cancers and diabetes, as well as cardiovascular disease. In addition, poor nutrition often leads to obesity, which remains an important risk factor for high blood pressure, heart attacks, and stroke.

Now we'll give you the fundamentals of proper nutrition, as they apply to cardiovascular health, and dispel the dietary myths listed at the beginning of this chapter. Then we'll give you some guidelines for setting up a safe, effective, and enjoyable eating plan to help you on your way toward a healthy heart and circulatory system.

The ABCs of Proper Nutrition

The human body requires about 40 different essential nutrients in order to carry out its functions and maintain its health. These nutrients include oxygen, water, protein, carbohydrates, fats, and a host of vitamins and minerals. The body receives oxygen from the air you breathe; without it, you could not survive for more than a few minutes. Although most of us take oxygen for granted, study after study proves that the more oxygen you supply to your body's cells—by breathing deeply and circulating more oxygen-rich blood during aerobic exercise—the better.

Water, which is found in most everything we eat and drink, is another substance we tend to take for granted. Water regulates body temperature, circulation and excretion, and aids in digestion. It bathes virtually all of our cells in moisture. Nevertheless, few of us drink the 64 ounces (8 glasses) of water our body needs every day to stay healthy.

The other 38 or so essential nutrients are found in the food we eat. What we call a "balanced" diet is one that contains the appropriate amount—not too little and not too much—of those nutrients on a daily basis. In addition, a balanced diet involves providing the right amount of calories—the energy value of food—to maintain proper body weight. (A calorie represents the amount of energy the body would need to burn in order to use up that bit of food; any excess energy is stored as fat.)

Most of us grew up with the idea that a balanced diet included equal amounts of four food groups: dairy, grains, meats, and fruits/vegetables. Recently, the United States Department of Agriculture (USDA) developed a new way of looking at our daily diet. Called the Food Pyramid, it organizes food types into a pyramid of multisized boxes. Each box represents a type of food and the proportion of the daily diet it should comprise.

Carbohydrates—from cereals, breads, and whole grains—form the base of the pyramid and should make up the bulk of a nutritious diet. At the much smaller tip of the triangle is fat; as you can see, fat should form a very small portion of your day's diet. In between are proteins, dairy products, and fruits and vegetables, all of which are to be eaten in varying proportions. Many people choose to obtain all the nutrients they need from a balanced diet, like the one described below and illustrated in the Food Pyramid. However, new evidence has surfaced about the role of antioxidants and other qualities of vitamins and minerals in the prevention and treatment of disease. In Chapter 5, we'll discuss this aspect of alternative medicine in more depth.

For now, let's take a look at the fundamentals of a healthy diet based on the Food Pyramid plan.

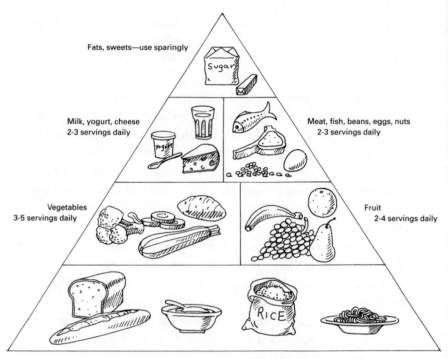

Fats, sweets—use sparingly

Milk, yogurt, cheese
2-3 servings daily

Meat, fish, beans, eggs, nuts
2-3 servings daily

Vegetables
3-5 servings daily

Fruit
2-4 servings daily

Bread, cereal, rice and pasta—6-11 servings daily

The Food Pyramid

Eating a wholesome diet is an important part of any
prevention and/or treatment plan—mainstream or alternative—for heart disease.
Although each individual has his or her own unique dietary needs,
the FDA Food Pyramid, pictured above, offers sound general guidelines
for a healthy, low-fat, high-carbohydrate diet.

The Truth about Cholesterol and Fat

Thanks to efforts by the American Heart Association and other health organizations, the word is out that consuming too much cholesterol and fat is bad for your health. And yet, there is still a great deal of misconception about what cholesterol is and how it affects your circulatory system. Which brings us to *Myth #1: Cholesterol causes heart disease.* In fact, all cholesterol is not bad, and cholesterol does not cause heart disease, at least not by itself.

HEART FACTS

Many people confuse fat and cholesterol, when, in fact, the two are quite different substances not always found together in the same food. For instance, three quarters of the calories in raw coconut come from saturated fat. But, like all plant foods, coconut is cholestrol-free.

Cholesterol is a lipid essential for a number of vital body processes, including nerve function, cell repair and reproduction, and the formation of various hormones, including estrogen and testosterone and the stress hormone cortisol. Because it is so important to the body, the human liver works very hard to create all the cholesterol we need every day to survive. In fact, the liver produces about 3,000 milligrams of new cholesterol in any 24-hour period, a quantity equivalent to the amount contained in 10 eggs.

And there's the rub: The body manufactures *all* the cholesterol it needs. Any cholesterol you consume is "extra" and can lead to health problems if there is enough of it circulating in the bloodstream. In addition, cholesterol-rich foods are frequently high in saturated fats (discussed below) and are often fried, leading to the conversion of the cholesterol to an activated, or dangerous, form.

Cholesterol travels through the bloodstream by combining with other lipids and certain proteins. When combined, these substances are called lipoproteins. One type of lipoprotein, called high-density lipoprotein (HDL), is beneficial to the body because it carries cholesterol away from the cells back to the liver, where it is then processed and finally eliminated from the body. HDL-cholesterol is known as the "good" cholesterol.

Another type of lipoprotein, however, is considered harmful to the body. Called low-density lipoprotein (LDL), this substance carries about two thirds of circulating cholesterol to the cells. This is often the "fat" we speak of when referring to the plaque that builds up and causes atherosclerosis. The relationship between these two kinds of lipoprotein determines the amount of cholesterol circulating through the bloodstream and, hence, an individual's risk of developing atherosclerosis.

Research indicates that LDL-cholesterol may become harmful only after it has been oxidized, or combined with oxygen. Oxidation occurs through a complicated chemical reaction in the body, a process that you may be able to prevent—or at least limit—if you eat plenty of foods rich in B vitamins, particularly vitamin B_6, vitamin B_{12}, and folic acid.

In foods, cholesterol is found primarily in animal products, such as meats and dairy products, which also tend to be high in fat and calories. In addition, cooking foods in a way that exposes them to oxygen and/or raises their temperature to high levels may increase the amount of harmful cholesterol that eventually reaches your bloodstream. In fact, hard- or soft-boiled and poached eggs do not appear to raise cholesterol levels in most individuals, while scrambled or fried eggs, the preparation of which exposes the cholesterol-rich yolks to both oxygen and high heat, may significantly raise cholesterol levels.

One of the most significant factors to consider when discussing the impact of cholesterol on heart disease is its relationship to the amount of fat in the diet. Research suggests that excess fat in the bloodstream may act as a trigger, stimulating the liver to produce more cholesterol, which then circulates in the bloodstream.

In fact, cholesterol is only one of several different forms of fat-like substances that may act in a harmful way in the body. Although we hear every day how bad fat is for us, the fact remains that we need to consume a little bit of fat—about the equivalent of one tablespoon—in order to survive, thus dispelling *Myth #2: All fat is bad.* Indeed, fats perform several vital functions in the body. They store energy, help to maintain healthy skin and hair, and carry fat-soluble vitamins (A, D, E, and K) through the bloodstream. They also provide the body with substances called essential fatty acids, which are the raw materials for several hormonelike compounds, including prostaglandins, which help regulate blood pressure, inflammation, and other body functions.

In general, there are three kinds of fats—saturated, monounsaturated, and polyunsaturated—that are found in varying amounts in all foods that contain fat. It helps to know which kind of fat you're eating, because different kinds of fat affect your cholesterol levels differently. Packaged foods are usually labeled by the fat that dominates in it, even though other kinds of fat may also be present.

Saturated fats are found in hydrogenated vegetable shortenings and in animal products such as whole milk, some cheeses, butter, meat, and cream. One way to recognize a saturated fat is that it is solid at room temperature. Processed peanut butter and margarine are two examples. Saturated fats are the fats to avoid; they tend to raise the level of cholesterol in the blood by 5 to 10 percent.

Monounsaturated fats, like peanut oil and olive oil, remain liquid at room temperature. These fats may actually work to lower LDL ("bad" cholesterol) levels in the bloodstream. Olive oil, in particular, may lower LDL levels while keeping HDL ("good" cholesterol) levels the same, a net benefit to the body. (Peanut oil, on the other hand, will lower both HDL and LDL, so the benefit to the body is less.)

Unsaturated fats, also called *polyunsaturated fats,* consist of liquid vegetable oils, like sunflower, corn, soybean, and sesame. Important dietary unsaturated fats also come from plants and fish. These fats may actually lower the amount of cholesterol in our bodies. Moreover, the polyunsaturated fats in fish oil, especially from cold-water fish such as salmon, contain a special kind of polyunsaturated fatty acid called omega-3, which the fish get from eating certain plants. Omega-3s offer an additional benefit: they make the blood less likely to clot, thus reducing the chances of artery blockage and heart attack.

Unfortunately, all fats are high in calories, and no matter how beneficial they might be to your blood lipid levels, they add excess pounds to your body if you eat too much of them. If you're like most Americans who have not adjusted your diet to reduce the fat you eat, you're probably consuming at least 37 percent of your daily calories in fat. By cutting down as much as possible on fat, you'll kill at least two birds with one dietary stone. First, by reducing fat you'll automatically reduce calories, helping you lose weight if you need to or maintain your weight while age slows your metabolism.

Second, and just as important, lowering your daily intake of all fatty foods will help you guard against the development of atherosclerosis and heart disease because you'll automatically reduce the amount of saturated fat you eat. Keep in mind that, even if you're not overweight, you may still be consuming too much cholesterol and fat, which then circulate through the bloodstream, damaging vessels along the way.

How much is too much? Prescriptions vary. The American Cancer Society suggests that no more than 30 percent of all calories consumed each day should come from fats and, further, that less than 10 percent of all caloric intake should come from saturated fat, up to 10 percent from polyunsaturated fats, and the remainder from monounsaturated fats.

Some health professionals advocate a much more dramatic decrease in fat. Dean Ornish, M.D., director of the effective "Opening Your Heart Program" at the University of California Medical Center, suggests reducing fat to less than 10 percent of your daily caloric intake. For the average adult male who eats about 2,500 calories a day, then, 250 calories or less should come from fat. Since each gram of fat contains 9 calories, an eating plan based on 10 percent fat content would allow about 27 grams of fat a day, the equivalent of what's contained in a single 4-ounce, untrimmed, broiled T-bone steak.

For some people, cutting back that much on fat is difficult. To many of us, fat tastes good, it gives food a certain "roundness" and smoothness we've learned to enjoy. In addition, fat takes longer to digest, and therefore gives us a feeling of fullness for longer periods of time. Finally, our busy lifestyles lend themselves to eating foods fried in oil, processed with saturated fats, and kept in fast-food heaters, all of which lead to a dangerous accumulation of harmful lipids in the blood. However, if you reduce the amount of fat in your diet, you'll be saving room for healthier foods, like grains, fruits, and vegetables, that can be every bit as tasty once your taste buds get used to them.

FAT AND CHOLESTEROL PRESCRIPTION

- Try to limit your daily fat intake to 10 to 20 percent of your daily caloric intake. If you eat 2,000 calories a day, only 200 to 400 of those calories should consist of calories derived from fat. (200 calories equals about 21 grams of fat.)
- Stay away from fat from animal sources such as whole milk, cheese, fatty meats, and poultry, which are more likely to contain saturated fats.
- Eat more fatty, cold-water fish, such as salmon, mackerel, halibut, tuna, and sardines. These have a protective effect on the arteries.
- Avoid hardened, hydrogenated oils such as margarine and processed foods.
- Use polyunsaturated oils (safflower, corn, etc.) in moderation. These oils should be kept refrigerated and fresh to avoid oxidation.
- Cook with olive, canola, or other monounsaturated oils, which will be less likely to oxidize.
- Broil or bake your foods. Don't fry them.
- Squirt 2 to 3 vitamin E capsules into each fresh bottle of oil to help preserve its freshness.
- Cook eggs with the yolks intact (hard- or soft-boiled or poached) to prevent cholesterol from becoming oxidized.

- Don't leave foods to warm for long periods of time.
- Many common foods have been found to lower blood lipids and/or raise good HDL-cholesterol. Eat more dried beans and legumes, apples and other fruits high in fiber called pectin, garlic and onions, oats and other grains high in soluble fiber, avocados, nonfat yogurt, black mushrooms, oysters, and almonds.
- Focus on lowering the fat, refined carbohydrates (see below), and processed foods in your diet, rather than on cholesterol.

Carbohydrates: The Body's Fuel

Carbohydrates form the large bottom end of the Food Pyramid. All plant material, including grains, fruits, and vegetables, contains some carbohydrates. Carbohydrates are the body's major source of energy. Once digested, they are broken down and either immediately used as fuel by the cells or stored in the liver or muscles for later use. When your body needs energy, it turns first to calories from carbohydrates.

There are three major types of carbohydrate—simple, complex, and dietary fiber. *Simple carbohydrates* are the sugars that come from fruits and vegetables, milk, and cane or beet. Table sugar, refined honey, and fruit sugar are all forms of simple carbohydrates. During the refining process, carbohydrates lose much of their nutritional value but retain their calories.

Complex carbohydrates, also known as starches, are found in bread, cereals, grains, pasta, fruits, and vegetables. Although the Food Pyramid includes separate sections for fruits and vegetables, they are really part of this larger group of carbohydrates.

Both simple and complex carbohydrates are easily digested and converted into glucose, the main fuel used by body cells for energy. However, complex carbohydrates are a better source of nutrition for the body for a number of reasons. First, complex carbohydrates are absorbed more slowly by the bloodstream because the process of digestion is more complicated. Simple carbohydrates—the sugars—

need less digestion and are therefore absorbed more quickly by the cells; any excess glucose gets stored more quickly as fat.

Second, foods made up of complex carbohydrates are also usually low in fat, high in dietary fiber, and come with a lot of nutritional extras. A slice of whole-wheat bread, for instance, not only contains carbohydrates, but also packs about 2 grams of protein, fiber, and several other nutritive substances, including riboflavin, thiamine, niacin, calcium, and iron. Simple carbohydrates, on the other hand, usually come in high-calorie, high-fat packages, like cookies and cakes.

Third, the problems with refined and simple carbohydrates go beyond their low nutrient value and propensity to turn into fat in the body. Sucrose, the most common form of sugar, is associated with higher rates of atherosclerosis and lipid levels, compared with the same calorie diet of starches. A high-sucrose diet is also associated with high insulin levels in the blood. Insulin is the hormone necessary for converting sugar into glucose, the body's fuel. High insulin levels are also implicated in arterial wall damage, and sugar increases the stickiness of platelets. In fact, there is good evidence that diets high in refined carbohydrates are more associated with heart disease than diets high in cholesterol. As if that weren't enough, high-sugar diets actually promote the excretion of valuable minerals such as chromium and magnesium.

An enduring rumor is *Myth #3: Carbohydrates make you fat.* In fact, they work to do just the opposite. If the carbohydrates you eat are complex carbohydrates, you are likely to lose, not gain, weight. If you consume too many simple carbohydrates, on the other hand, you're bound to put on pounds.

Dietary fiber is the third type of carbohydrate and is present in whole grains, fruits, and vegetables. Also called roughage, fiber is not broken down by human digestive enzymes and therefore is not absorbed into the bloodstream. Although it provides no nutrients, fiber helps aid in digestion and helps keep the digestive tract clean and clear.

Dietary fiber, particularly that found in fruits, also helps to lower blood pressure, although exactly how it does so is still poorly understood. It may work by lowering the amount of insulin circulating in the blood. It might also help the body to excrete more sodium.

There are two kinds of fiber, insoluble and soluble. Insoluble fiber acts like a sponge, absorbing many times its weight in water. As it moves through the digestive tract, it pushes food along with it and out of the body through waste elimination. This process may also help to excrete substances known as bile acids, which are cholesterol-containing digestive enzymes formed by the liver. Soluble fiber, on the other hand, appears to help reduce blood fat levels and, in some cases, increase HDL levels as well. For instance, oat bran and rice bran contain a type of soluble fiber that seems to bind up cholesterol in the digestive tract. Carrots, apples, and grapefruits are all high in pectin, another kind of soluble fiber shown to lower LDL and raise HDL.

CARBOHYDRATE PRESCRIPTION

- According to the American Heart Association and the USDA, you should consume about 20 to 30 grams of fiber every day. A ½ cup of brown rice contains 2.4 grams of fiber, a ½ cup of kidney beans about 7 grams, and a large pear almost 6 grams of fiber.
- Complex carbohydrates, consisting of whole grains, vegetables, and fruits should make up about 50 to 60 percent of your daily calories.
- Choose foods high in soluble fiber.
- Avoid simple sugars (including corn syrup, dextrose, and fructose, frequently added to processed foods) and simple carbohydrates (white flour products).

Fruits and Vegetables

Although occupying separate sections in the USDA's Food Pyramid, fruit and vegetables are often combined in discussions about nutrition because they contain many of the same nutrients and provide us with the same overall health benefits. Fruits and vegetables are, with a few exceptions, low in fat and calories, high in fiber, and chock full of vitamins and minerals. In fact, fruits and vegetables provide about 92 percent of the vitamin C and half of the vitamin A in the nation's food supply, while contributing just 9 percent of the calories.

Most fruit is higher in sugar and calories than most vegetables. On the other hand, some vegetables contain such high levels of complex carbohydrates that they are classified as starches. These starchy vegetables include potatoes, corn, peas, and some types of beans (black, fava, kidney), among others. That is not to say that these foods are not good for you. In fact, starchy vegetables are among the best sources of fiber and vitamins available. However, compared with leafy green vegetables, like collard greens, kale, and spinach, which also have a high fiber content, starchy vegetables are much higher in calories.

Many alternative practitioners recommend eating as many plant-based foods as possible and reducing, if not eliminating, meat and animal foods in the diet. As you'll see in the following section, vegetarian diets can provide all the nutrients you need without the fats and other chemicals that come with animal products. Eating plenty of grains, fresh fruits, and vegetables—foods that by nature are whole and unprocessed—will provide you with more fiber, less fat, decreased sugar, and more nutrients.

Protein: The Building Block of Life

The term protein comes from the Greek word *protos*, which means first and foremost. Indeed, proteins are found in every body cell, constitute the second most plentiful substance in the body of a normal-weight person, and make up about one fifth of a normal adult's body weight. Protein is the major component of our muscles, organs, bones, skin, antibodies, some hormones, and virtually all enzymes (substances that speed up the rate of biochemical actions).

Protein molecules are made up of organic compounds called amino acids. There are 23 amino acids; of these, the body can manufacture all but 8. These 8 are called "essential amino acids" and they must be obtained from the diet. Meat, egg white, milk, and other animal products are rich in dietary protein. Plant material—specifically grains, legumes (certain beans and peas), and certain vegetables—also contains varying amounts of proteins, but no one plant source provides all of the essential amino acids in the right amount for human use. Such plant-derived foods can nonetheless be excellent sources of protein, if eaten in combinations that supply all of the essential amino acids.

Although it may take a bit more research to discover which combinations of grains and vegetables make up a complete protein source, many health professionals are urging their patients with heart disease to increase their plant-protein intake while cutting back on animal protein. Although animal products appear to offer the best balance of protein, they are also often filled with saturated fats and calories. A one-ounce slice of cheddar cheese, for instance, contains 7 grams of protein, but more than 70 percent of its calories come from fat. Even extra lean hamburger, broiled well-done, derives about 52 percent of its calories from fat. Which brings us to *Myth #4: Extra protein makes you strong.* Just the opposite is true: eating more protein, especially animal protein, will not add to strength, muscle development, or athletic prowess. Excess protein is usually stored as fat.

Furthermore, high-protein diets (like the typical American diet) lead to the loss of calcium in the kidneys, which encourages the weakening of bones known as osteoporosis. Animal proteins (like casein found in dairy products) tend to increase cholesterol, while vegetable protein foods (such as soybeans) contain substances called saponins, which lower cholesterol. Dairy products, in fact, present another problem. Homogenized milk is strongly associated with atherosclerosis, even the 1 percent, low-fat kind. There is experimental work suggesting that a toxic enzyme called xanthine oxidase is present in homogenized milk (though not in skim milk) and this enzyme may irritate the inner arterial walls.

You might be surprised how easy it is to obtain all the protein you need from foods other than red meat or eggs. Four ounces of pasta, for instance, provides about 20 percent of the Recommended Daily Allowance (RDA) for protein, as much as two large eggs.

PROTEIN PRESCRIPTION

Most of your protein should be from nonanimal sources such as beans. Luckily, we need to consume a relatively small amount of protein to meet all our needs. Protein makes up about 25 percent of the typical American diet, almost twice the recommended 12 to 15 percent.

Dairy Products: Calcium Providers

The final portion of the Food Pyramid to be discussed is devoted to dairy products, namely milk, yogurt, and cheese. These foods contain large amounts of an essential mineral, calcium, which plays an important role in the cardiovascular system. Calcium is necessary for proper clotting of the blood and also helps to maintain blood pressure by controlling contraction of the muscles in blood vessel walls and heart tissue. Calcium is also essential to the health of your bones, teeth, and nails.

Although the Food Pyramid recommends just two servings—about 2 cups of milk or 2 ounces of cheese—every day, most of us neglect this aspect of our diet, partly because dairy products also tend to be rather high in fat and calories. To avoid consuming too much fat, you should choose skim versions of these products. If you have trouble digesting milk (a condition known as lactose intolerance) or simply do not enjoy dairy products, you can get calcium from other foods, including sardines and leafy green vegetables, such as turnip greens and collard greens, and broccoli.

If you find you are unable to meet your calcium needs through your diet, there are several types of calcium supplements available. Discuss which type of supplement might be best for you with your physician or alternative practitioner and see Chapter 5 for more information.

DAIRY PRESCRIPTION
- Your goal should be to get 1,000 milligrams or more of calcium each day, an amount that can be found in 2 cups of skim milk or skim yogurt.
- Work on adding nondairy sources of calcium to your diet.

Customize Your Eating Plan

Although we've given you some guidelines to follow in planning a diet for a healthy cardiovascular system, it is essential that you discuss your own needs with your alternative practitioner. One of the benefits of choosing natural medicine over mainstream therapy is the very personal and individual approach it takes to health and disease. Let your practitioner use his or her knowledge of this aspect of natural medicine to help you create an eating plan that's right for you.

Getting Out the Toxins

In addition to the foods we eat, there are at least three other substances commonly consumed by Americans on a regular basis: cigarette smoke, coffee, and alcohol, all of which are related to

Tips for Healthy Eating

What you eat can go a long way
in helping you keep your heart healthy.
Try these simple tips:

- Eat more high-protein plant foods like grains, legumes, nuts, and seeds.
- Buy seasonal foods. Vegetables and fruits grown out of season often have to be induced to grow with chemicals and artificial light, which may have negative health effects.
- Choose frozen over canned fruits and vegetables if fresh produce is unavailable. Canned produce usually has been processed more than its frozen counterparts.
- Avoid food additives and preservatives, like aspartame, Red Dye #2, monosodium glutamate, nitrites, and sulfur dioxide, found in most processed foods. Eat more fresh, whole foods.
- Read food labels carefully to find out the quantities of essential nutrients, fat, and additives contained in the product.
- Eat a variety of foods to keep your taste buds satisfied and to increase the nutrients you consume on a daily basis.

cardiovascular disease. At the end of this chapter, we'll explore how to eliminate another risk factor related to nutrition and cardiovascular disease: obesity.

Cigarette smoking. It may seem odd to include information about smoking in a chapter on nutrition, but when you think about it, smoking introduces substances into the blood just like eating does.

According to the United States Surgeon General, cigarette smoking is the single most preventable cause of heart disease and is responsible for at least 30 percent of all heart-disease-related deaths annually. The famous Framingham Heart Study found that men who smoke have a tenfold increased risk of death from cardiac arrest over those men who do not smoke; among women smokers, the mortality rate is five-fold over women nonsmokers.

The dangers from cigarette smoke start with just one cigarette a day and increase with every cigarette smoked: Smoking one to ten cig-arettes per day doubles the mortality rate from heart disease. Smok-ing ten to twenty cigarettes per day increases the mortality another 25 percent. And smoking more than two packs a day triples the death rate. Smokers have a stunning 70 percent higher rate of death from heart disease than nonsmokers.

There are some 4,000 substances identified in cigarette smoke—some highly toxic and carcinogenic. Nicotine is cigarette smoke's main active ingredient. When you inhale a cigarette, nicotine imme-diately enters your bloodstream and reaches your brain within six sec-onds, where more than 15 percent of it is absorbed. Nicotine is a stimulant. When it reaches your brain, it signals your adrenal glands to release norepinephrine and epinephrine, which increase your blood pressure. Your heart beats faster, it pumps more blood, and your arteries work harder to push the blood through your body.

In addition to directly causing an increase in heart and vessel activ-ity, cigarette smoking also contributes to the acceleration of atheroscle-rosis. Nicotine, as well as other products of cigarette smoke, raises the amount of fats and cholesterol circulating in the bloodstream, which, as you know, form plaque on artery walls. In fact, cigarette smoking has been shown to raise the level of LDLs by as much as 10 percent.

Atherosclerosis is accelerated by another ingredient of cigarette smoke—carbon monoxide—as well. Carbon monoxide damages the cells that form the inner linings of arterial walls, making them more susceptible to plaque buildup.

To make matters worse, carbon monoxide is carried through the bloodstream by the same blood component, hemoglobin, that transports oxygen. The more carbon monoxide in the bloodstream, therefore, the less oxygen is being carried to the vital organs, including the heart. Cigarette smoking also causes chemical changes in the blood itself, causing it to become more sticky. This stickiness can result in the formation of large blood clots, which can cause both strokes and heart attacks.

Cigarette Prescription
- If you smoke, stop as soon as you can. There are several programs and methods that have been developed by the American Heart Association, the American Lung Association, and other groups that might be of help.
- Talk to your practitioner about natural substances, like chlorophyll, and the amino acid L-glutamine that may help you in your effort to beat the habit.
- Acupuncture, hypnosis, and biofeedback have all been used successfully in "stop smoking" programs, but the first step is to sit down and really convince yourself that you want to stop. You can try any of these therapies. Stopping because someone tells you it's bad will not work.

Coffee. Drinking more than 3 cups of coffee per day has been shown to elevate blood lipids. And above 5 cups per day is strongly associated with heart attacks. This is not true of tea and colas, so the caffeine is not totally responsible. Blood pressure also rises with this amount of coffee drinking. So does the incidence of heart-rhythm disturbances. To date, it is unclear whether decaffeinated coffee is any less potentially harmful.

Coffee Prescription
- Limit coffee drinking to 3 or fewer cups per day.
- Switching to decaf might be prudent.
- If you must have a caffeinated beverage, switch to tea.

Alcohol. Recent studies have shown that moderate drinking—defined as one or two drinks a day—may have *beneficial* effects on the cardiovascular system. This phenomenon has been nicknamed the "French paradox" because the health benefits of alcohol consumption are especially evident among the French, who have far lower mortality rates due to heart disease than do Americans—despite the fact that they eat a diet equal or higher in fat levels.

A key difference between the American and French diets appears to be in the amount of alcohol—specifically red wine—the two cultures imbibe. Red wine apparently affects the cardiovascular system by working to increase the levels of HDL, the "good" cholesterol. By what mechanism this occurs is still not completely understood, but scientists believe that certain chemicals in alcohol, known as phenols, help metabolize lipids and more quickly remove them from the bloodstream. In essence, then, *Myth #5—Alcohol is always harmful*—is dispelled.

In fact, people who consume one to two drinks per day tend to have slightly lower blood pressures than those who abstain from drinking completely. This suggests that moderate alcohol intake may have a favorable effect on blood pressure.

It is possible to have too much of a good thing, however. The more alcohol someone consumes after the second drink, the more he or she risks damaging the cardiovascular system. The relationship between heavy drinking—more than two or three drinks a day—and high blood pressure has been well documented. Several studies, including the Framingham Heart Study, the Los Angeles Heart Study, and the Chicago Western Electric Study, showed that people who have histories of long-term, heavy drinking had significantly higher blood pressures than those people who were light drinkers or abstainers.

If you have high blood pressure, then, it is best that you keep your drinking to a minimum. In addition to its direct effects on the blood pressure system, alcohol interacts poorly with many blood pressure medications. If you are taking medication, make sure you discuss drinking any alcohol with your doctor.

Alcohol Prescription
- If you enjoy a cocktail before dinner or a glass of wine or two with your meal, feel free to continue this pleasurable and apparently harmless habit.
- If you are unable to handle alcohol physically or emotionally, if you have a family history of alcoholism, or if you simply don't like to drink, the risks of alcohol far outweigh the benefits and you should not feel pressured to partake.

Losing Weight

Obesity is a major risk factor for cardiovascular disease of all types. As many as 40 percent of all Americans are obese, or 20 percent over their ideal weight. Although losing weight—and keeping it off—can be very difficult for many of us, it is *essential* if we want to maintain our health.

Before we discuss how to lose weight, we should talk about how we put on extra pounds in the first place. Why do some people become overweight and others remain slim, even while appearing to eat the same amounts of food? It appears that genetics, individual metabolism, and a whole slew of other factors combine to determine someone's propensity to gain or lose weight. Like high blood pressure and heart disease, obesity is a disorder that goes hand-in-hand with other diseases—especially diabetes and atherosclerosis—that also run in families and that also predispose someone to heart disease.

At the heart of the matter, however, is a simple formula. To lose weight, you must burn off more calories than you consume. Eating any kind of food—even those we deem most healthful, such as fruits and vegetables—can cause you to gain weight, if you eat more calories than you burn off. The number of calories an individual needs to meet energy requirements depends on several factors, including age, weight, and level of exercise.

In addition, *what* you eat matters just as much as *how much* you eat. Indeed, all foods are not created equal: If two people eat the same weight of food in a day, but one person takes in 60 percent of her food in the form of complex carbohydrates while the other consumes her calories in the form of fat, the two will most likely end up with very different body shapes and weights.

Why? First, complex carbohydrates are used more efficiently than fat and are far less likely to be stored in the body. Experiments at the University of Massachusetts Medical School, for example, suggest that if you consume 100 excess carbohydrate calories, 23 of those calories will be used to simply process the food, and only 77 of them will end up being stored as fat. But it appears that only 3 calories are burned in the processing and storing of 100 fat calories.

Second, and most important, a gram of fat provides more than twice the calories of a gram of carbohydrates: 9 calories as compared with 4. That's why one ounce of potato chips—processed with fat and totaling more than 160 calories—is more fattening than one ounce of baked potato, which contains about 30 calories and no fat at all.

Finally, as we have seen before, all carbohydrates are not alike. A diet high in sugar and white flour (simple carbohydrates) will encourage fat storage. It will also increase hunger by increasing the amount of insulin circulating in your body.

CONSTRUCTING A HEALTHY EATING PLAN

The best way to eat well and maintain a healthy weight—or to lose weight if necessary—is to eat relatively small portions of a wide variety of foods and to exercise.

Fad diets that promise rapid weight loss and concentrate on eating just a few select foods are dangerous for many reasons. By concentrating solely on losing pounds and not on learning proper nutrition, you'll most likely fall back into the same kinds of bad eating habits that made you heavy in the first place. This kind of seesaw effect is both dangerous and counterproductive. Rapid weight loss puts an extraordinary strain on the cardiovascular system and also

A Healthy Eating Plan

The following portions of
protein, carbohydrates, fruits, vegetables,
breads, dairy products, and
fat will provide you with about 1,300
calories per day, enough for the
average adult American to lose a healthy
1 to 2 pounds per week.

- 4 to 6 ounces of lean protein (chicken, turkey, fish, lentils, dried peas, sprouts and grains, egg whites; avoid red meat, pork, whole eggs, and nuts, which have high amounts of fat and/or cholesterol)
- 4 or more cups of fresh (or fresh-frozen, without sauce) vegetables
- 3 servings of medium-sized fruit
- 4 to 6 servings of starches, each containing no more than 80 calories each (bread, English muffins, pasta, cereal, potatoes, rice, popcorn)
- Two 8-ounce servings of skim milk, nonfat yogurt, or low-fat cottage cheese
- No more than 2 tablespoons of fat

It is important that you discuss your
eating plan with your alternative practitioner.
He or she may have further
recommendations based on the clinical
exam he or she gives you.

changes the body's metabolic rate, forever lowering the number of calories your body needs to maintain vital functions. That's why people find it difficult to lose weight again after crash dieting. Also, once the body forms a fat cell, it can be shrunk but never eliminated.

Take another look at the Food Pyramid. By adapting proper portion control, you can use the pyramid to develop a safe, healthy, and effective eating plan to lose weight and thus relieve yourself of *Myth #6: Counting calories is the only effective way to lose weight.* The adaptation of a plan recommended by the American Heart Association, outlined on page 73, replaces the often tedious struggle of counting calories and "dieting" with the more natural approach of portion control and food variety. Notice the inclusion of both complex carbohydrates and some lean protein; a diet with complex carbohydrates alone can lead to fatigue and irritability.

Carefully watching what you eat—and reducing the amount of sugar-filled or fatty foods in your diet—may feel like a punishment, especially at first. With time, however, you may be surprised at how much you enjoy the taste of delicious, healthful food. Moreover, as the pounds drop away, you just may discover that you have more energy than you ever dreamed you had. In fact, even before you lose weight, your new commitment to a healthy lifestyle may prompt you to add another important component to any cardiovascular fitness plan: exercise. In Chapter 6, you'll learn the principles of safe, effective activity and all about what it can do for your heart and blood pressure. In the meantime, in Chapter 5 we'll talk more about the role of vitamins and minerals in preventing and treating cardiovascular disease.

"*If anything is sacred, the human body is sacred.*"

Walt Whitman

5

Vitamins and Minerals

....

$\mathcal{V}$itamins and minerals are substances that your body needs to perform a wide variety of functions. For much of the 20th century, it was widely believed that most Americans derived all the vitamins and minerals they required from the foods they consumed. Recent evidence, however, suggests that we may need to take in additional vitamins and minerals for three reasons: First, the average American diet is packed with calorie-rich but nutritionally insubstantial food. In other words, we do not eat enough whole grains, fruits, and vegetables to obtain even the minimum amounts of some of the vitamins and minerals our bodies need to function properly.

Second, our modern lifestyles and environment use up nutrients in quantities beyond what even the healthiest diet may replace. For instance, pollutants deplete the body's quantity of antioxidants, stress lowers our supply of vitamins B and C, food dyes and preservatives block vitamin B_6 and folate, and heavy metals in the soil, sea, and even our dental fillings may interfere with our trace mineral nutrition. A diet high in protein, sugar, fats, and sodium also promotes the excretion of valuable nutrients. Your body has to use up these essential substances just to digest and extract energy from this kind of diet.

Third, it appears that the conventional standard of vitamin and mineral requirements, set by the Food and Nutrition Board of the National Research Council, may be woefully understated. Called the U.S. Recommended Daily Allowance (RDA), this standard has undergone several revisions since it was first established in the 1940s. It is currently undergoing another update in the wake of new evidence suggesting that taking far larger amounts of certain vitamins, called antioxidants, may help prevent a myriad of diseases, including cancer and heart disease.

Furthermore, as practitioners of alternative medicine have known for centuries, each individual has different nutritional requirements, based on his or her own particular metabolism, lifestyle, and medical imperatives. This principle was stated by the famous scientist Dr. Roger Williams as "biochemical individuality," and it is spreading, slowly but steadily, through the halls of mainstream medicine. It may well affect how we think about nutritional requirements in the future.

For now, it's important for every American concerned about cardiovascular disease to be aware of how vitamins and minerals work to maintain body functions and, then, how they affect the heart, the blood, and the blood vessels.

The Role of Vitamins and Minerals

Vitamins are organic substances found in plants and animals. Generally speaking, the body cannot manufacture vitamins and so we must obtain them through the diet or through the use of supplements. There are approximately 14 vitamins considered vital to life, and several other nutrients whose roles are just beginning to be recognized.

Each vitamin carries out specific functions, and the lack of a certain vitamin can lead to subtle biochemical problems or, in extreme deficiencies, to severe diseases. For instance, low vitamin D intake can lead to problems in calcium metabolism such as osteoporosis and, in its severe childhood form, can lead to the degenerative bone condition called rickets. Some vitamins, such as E and B6, affect all cells and functions in the body without having a specific deficiency disease associated with them.

Minerals, on the other hand, are inorganic substances that are basic constituents of the earth's crust. Carried into the soil and groundwater, they are taken up by plants and consumed by humans. Of the more than 60 different minerals in the body, there are 22 that are considered essential. Seven of these, including calcium, chloride, magnesium, phosphorus, potassium, sodium, and sulfur, are considered major minerals. Others, called trace minerals, are found in tiny amounts in the body, but their importance belies their small quantities.

Several nutritive substances are especially important when discussing cardiovascular health. They include the antioxidants (vitamins C, E, and beta-carotene and minerals zinc and selenium), vitamin B_6, niacin, sodium, potassium, and magnesium. At the end of the chapter, we'll give you some suggestions on how much of these vitamins and minerals may be beneficial to you. However, it is important to realize that each and every individual has different requirements. You must discuss your own personal needs with your alternative practitioner and/or a licensed nutritionist.

Now let's look at the role different vitamins and minerals play in maintaining your cardiovascular health.

Antioxidants. Studies reveal that certain vitamins, particularly vitamins C, E, and beta-carotene (a precursor of vitamin A), may be especially helpful in fighting disease. These vitamins have the ability to destroy certain harmful molecules in the body called free radicals and therefore prevent them from oxidizing or damaging the tissues.

One study on the role of antioxidants in heart disease was done by Joann Manson, M.D., and Charles Hennekens, M.D., of Harvard

Medical School and Brigham and Women's Hospital in Boston. After monitoring the diet and vitamin use of 87,000 nurses for more than a decade, the investigators found that the women whose vitamin E consumption was in the upper 20 percent had a 35 percent lower risk of heart disease, even when all other factors, like smoking, blood pressure, and cholesterol, were taken into account. Those whose beta-carotene consumption was in the upper 20 percent had a 22 percent lower risk of heart disease.

These vitamins have a number of beneficial effects in the fight against heart disease. Vitamin E is known to make platelets less sticky, thus protecting against the formation of harmful clots. It also increases HDL levels and protects the other antioxidants. Vitamin E has been used successfully to treat claudication, a problem of atherosclerotic plaque blocking the arteries to the legs.

Vitamin C has a wide range of beneficial effects, including aiding in the breakdown of fats and in the conversion of cholesterol to bile acids (and thus lowering cholesterol levels in the blood). It, too, helps decrease platelet stickiness. Vitamin C also strengthens the arterial walls against damage, increases HDL levels, and lowers the mortality from heart attacks.

The mineral selenium is also considered an antioxidant, because it is necessary for the proper function of the important antioxidant enzyme glutathione peroxidase (which renders harmless the oxidized lipids called lipid peroxides). Low selenium levels are associated with high rates of atherosclerotic heart disease. This situation is made worse if vitamin E levels are low as well. Selenium also makes the platelets less sticky.

Zinc is also needed for antioxidant enzymes to function, and also makes platelets less sticky. However, in moderate-to-high doses (above 50 milligrams a day), it will lower HDLs (the good cholesterol). This is probably due to the fact that zinc competes with copper, which seems to aid in lowering cholesterol and strengthening the connective tissue in the artery wall. Thus, people taking zinc supplementation for various reasons (prostate, skin, and immune function, for example) should always take copper as well.

Nutrients involved in high blood pressure. The major minerals sodium, potassium, calcium, and magnesium all play roles in heart disease and in high blood pressure. *Sodium*, a metallic element found in nearly everything we eat, is directly related to high blood pressure, a major contributor to heart disease. Sodium affects blood pressure in two ways: First, it affects the kidneys' ability to excrete fluids, thereby raising the body's fluid volume; as fluid levels rise, so too does blood pressure. Second, it stimulates the nervous system, causing it to release norepinephrine and epinephrine—the "fight-or-flight" hormones—which also raise blood pressure.

If consumed in large quantities over time, sodium may raise blood pressure too high, although most people who eat too much salt excrete it through urination or perspiration. (Sodium is a major component of table salt.) Those who are salt-sensitive, on the other hand, tend to retain salt and fluids and thus raise their blood pressures. Salt sensitivity is believed to be genetically determined and linked to low levels of renin, a hormone secreted by the kidney that raises blood pressures. Researchers believe that about half of all people who have high blood pressure are salt-sensitive; among African-Americans, the percentage is even higher—as high as 70 to 80 percent.

No one has ever developed an effective way to distinguish between those people who are salt-sensitive and those who aren't. For that reason most experts recommend that we *all* decrease the amount of salt we consume. And we consume quite a lot. Although the actual physiological need for sodium may be as low as 220 milligrams a day, most of us consume over twenty times that amount, or 5,000 milligrams each day.

The main source of sodium in the average American's diet is sodium chloride, commonly known as table salt. In that form, it is used as a spice and as a preservative and is found in greater or lesser amounts in nearly everything we eat. One of the first steps you should take to reduce the amount of salt you eat is to throw away your salt shaker— not just the salt you put on your food at the table, but also what you use to spice food while you're cooking.

The second step in your quest for salt reduction may be a bit more difficult: Avoid processed foods (including canned soups, fruits, and vegetables and frozen dinners that are not specifically labeled "low sodium"), fast-food restaurants, and snack foods. It is essential that you check food labels for sodium content: Even foods that don't taste salty may be loaded with the stuff. Breakfast cereals are notoriously salty, for instance, as is American cheese and tuna fish.

You may find at first that reducing your salt intake is difficult and that you miss the way salt makes food taste. However, the longer you go without it, the less you'll miss it—and the more you'll savor the true flavors of food. To perk up the natural flavor of food, try using spices and herbs such as tarragon, pepper, basil, oregano, cumin, parsley, ginger, and the list goes on. Sea salt (found in health food stores) consists of other minerals besides sodium, and may be a good substitute used in moderation. There are hundreds of low-salt cookbooks available should you want to further experiment with herbs, wine, and other cooking methods to help spice up life-after-salt.

A chemical essential for muscle contraction and other body functions, *potassium* also plays a role in helping the kidneys eliminate sodium from the body. Some doctors recommend potassium supplements to help lower blood pressure, particularly when combined with magnesium. Potassium is found in high quantities in oranges and orange juice, peanut butter, dried peas and beans, yogurt, molasses, and meat.

Is it possible to prevent cardiovascular disease by consuming more potassium? Probably not. But, luckily, potassium is most often found in food low in sodium, so that when you reduce your intake of sodium, you often automatically increase your intake of potassium. Once you cut down on the amount of sodium you eat, the naturally high levels of potassium in your diet may have more of an impact on lowering your blood pressure. Please be aware that the use of potassium supplements is highly controversial, since too much potassium (hyperkalemia) can cause serious illness. Discuss whether or not you need extra potassium with your physician or alternative practitioner before taking supplements.

Magnesium is a mineral that helps regulate nerve and muscle function, including normal heart rhythm. The discovery of magnesium's role in proper heart and circulatory function may be the single greatest breakthrough in nutritional approaches to cardiac care. Magnesium is a mineral that works in tandem with calcium. Calcium is responsible for the contraction of muscles and the firing of nerves; and magnesium is responsible for the relaxation of muscles and nerves. In fact, magnesium is a natural calcium-channel blocker functioning much like the calcium-channel blocker drugs that are commonly used in high blood pressure, heart failure, and angina. Heart muscle has *fifteen times* as much magnesium as other muscle in the body.

But magnesium's role goes beyond this important area. It is also necessary for the exchange of oxygen in the tissues, it lowers LDL and raises HDL, it tones down the sympathetic nervous system, in a manner similar to the cardiac drugs called beta-blockers, and it slows down the processes that lead to atherosclerosis, platelet aggregation, and fibrin clotting in the arterial wall. Finally, magnesium frequently helps vitamin B$_6$ carry out its all-important functions.

Considering all that magnesium does, it's no wonder that multiple studies have linked low magnesium levels with atherosclerosis, heart attacks, high blood pressure, arrhythmias, and even mitral valve prolapse syndrome. There is even some data suggesting that prenatal magnesium deficiency is responsible for infant deaths due to cardiovascular causes.

Magnesium is found in complex carbohydrates, especially wheat bran, raw leafy green vegetables, nuts, and bananas, among other foods. However, for those of us who have atherosclerosis or some other type of cardiovascular disease, it is difficult to get enough of the mineral through the diet. To make matters worse, the modern emphasis on calcium and vitamin D has the effect of increasing the body's need for magnesium to balance the calcium. Many nutritional practitioners suggest a 1:1 calcium:magnesium ratio rather than the conventional 2:1 ratio. There is even some convincing evidence that magnesium is as important as calcium in the prevention of osteoporosis.

In addition to the nutritive substances discussed so far, there are several others believed to play a large role in the prevention and treatment of cardiovascular disease:

Calcium. Calcium, like its fellow minerals, has been shown to lower blood lipids and make platelets less sticky. It also seems to help lower blood pressure, probably by lowering the hormone called parathyroid hormone. This hormone moves calcium into the muscles, helping to enhance muscle contraction of the arterial wall. As mentioned above, calcium works best when balanced with magnesium.

Chromium. This mineral is woefully deficient in U.S. soils and thus in our diets. Even when eating the right kinds of food, it is difficult for us to obtain the right amount of chromium, which is necessary for blood sugar metabolism. Also, chromium is associated with high HDL- and low LDL-cholesterol levels, and has been shown in animals to slow and even reverse plaque formation.

Vitamin B₆. This vitamin has been shown to lower cholesterol, and lessen platelet stickiness, as well as help to bring oxygen to the heart muscle. Perhaps its greatest importance may be related to the theory of homocysteine buildup. This theory says that this substance, which is created when the amino acid methionine is metabolized, irritates the arterial wall if it is not eliminated. The theory also says that this buildup of homocysteine occurs more commonly than we think. Vitamin B₆, along with folic acid, is instrumental in converting homocysteine to a harmless by-product.

Niacin (vitamin B₃). Niacin may be effective in lowering blood lipids and increasing HDL-cholesterol. According to a 1986 article in the *Journal of the American Medical Association*, niacin is the "first drug to be used when dietary intervention fails" to lower high cholesterol levels. Using niacin to treat heart disease may result in serious side effects, however, and should be done only under the care of an experienced practitioner.

Omega-3 fatty acids. These oils, which come from cold-water fish and are present in flaxseed oil, lower blood lipid levels and prevent platelets from becoming sticky. However, care must be taken to prevent the oils from becoming rancid, at which time they become harmful free radicals. Keep flaxseed oil refrigerated and broil—do not fry—fish.

L-cysteine. This amino acid is a potent free radical scavenger.

L-taurine. Similar in function to magnesium, this amino acid improves the relaxation of nerve and muscle tissue, and has a demonstrated positive effect on arrhythmias and on congestive heart failure.

It's also possible that it could help in preventing heart attacks.

Choline and lecithin. These accessory B vitamins frequently occur along with cholesterol in nature (the egg yolk, for instance, is high in lecithin) and are known to lower blood lipids and increase HDL at the same time.

The next group of nutrients are synthesized in the body and therefore should be found in adequate amounts. However, as we have discussed above, the modern lifestyle frequently leads to deficiencies in important body components.

L-carnitine. This amino acid exists in high concentration in heart muscle, where it is crucial in the oxygenation and metabolism of cardiac tissue. Replenishing the heart carnitine concentration has been shown to improve circulation, reduce angina, improve treadmill tolerance, diminish cardiac arrhythmias, and help cardiomyopathies (abnormalities of heart muscle function).

Coenzyme-Q-10 (Co-Q-10). Derived from the B vitamin pantothenic acid, this substance carries energy through the tissues and is essential in the function of the cell mitochondria. Mitochondria are the cells' little energy factories. Low levels of Co-Q-10 are associated with almost all cardiac diseases, including angina, high blood pressure, mitral valve prolapse, and congestive heart failure. Examinations of heart muscle tissue routinely show 50 to 75 percent less Co-Q-10 in people with these illnesses. Even more important, the substance has been used successfully to treat heart disease and angina, high blood pressure, arrhythmias, and cardiomyopathies. Co-Q-10 lowers blood lipids while increasing HDL.

Chondroitin sulfate. This relatively unknown nutrient is a constituent of the arterial cell wall, and seems to bind LDL, preventing it from attaching to the plaque that is already there. It also has anticlotting properties, and aids in wound healing.

NUTRIENT PRESCRIPTION

Each and every human being is unique and thus has a distinct set of nutritional requirements. It is essential that you discuss your own needs with your physician and/or alternative practitioner before you take vitamin and mineral supplements.

Nutrients are best used in combinations with one another; otherwise, other deficiencies can be produced. Also, several nutrients are associated with side effects. In general, a nutrient program using doses above those recommended here should be followed only under the supervision of an experienced practitioner. Please note that all dosages given below are per day.

- *Vitamin A/beta-carotene*: 15,000 international units (IU), preferably beta-carotene. If using vitamin A, use the water-soluble palmitate form, which does not accumulate as easily in the liver.
- *Vitamin C*: 250–3,000 milligrams (mg) have been used safely. Please note that the higher the dose, the more risk there is of stomach irritation.
- *Vitamin D*: 400 IU.
- *Vitamin E*: 200–800 IU. Vitamin E is one of the few vitamins for which the natural form (called D-alpha-tocopherol) is clearly superior to the synthetic form (called DL-alpha-tocopherol). Caution: Doses of vitamin E in excess of 1,200 IU a day may increase blood pressure.
- *Vitamin B Complex*: 25–100 mg in a time-release tablet, or smaller amounts taken several times a day adding up to this level.
- *Vitamin B_6*: 10–50 mg per day have been found to have positive effects in the treatment of cardiovascular disease.
- *Vitamin B_3 (niacin)*: Niacin causes flushing, and niacin therapy should be initiated slowly. About 100 mg taken with meals is recommended at the start, gradually increasing the dose under supervision. Doses shown to lower cholesterol range from 3,000 to 6,000 mg. Please note: A new form of niacin, called inositol hexaniacinate may have the same positive effects as vitamin B_3 but without the side effects. Talk to your doctor or nutritionist.
- *Sodium*: Diet should contain 2 grams of sodium or *less* per day.

- *Potassium*: Dietary recommendations call for up to 5,500 mg. Potassium supplements, usually in 99 mg doses, can be taken several times per day.
- *Calcium*: 1,000 mg, increased to 1,500 in pregnant, nursing, and postmenopausal women. Good forms of calcium are lactate, gluconate, and citrate.
- *Magnesium*: Magnesium should be balanced one for one with calcium, especially in individuals with heart problems. Doses of magnesium up to 600–800 mg can be used safely, usually as citrate, gluconate, aspartate, or chelate.
- *Zinc*: 25–30 mg. Chelate and picolinate are good forms of zinc.
- *Copper*: 2 mg should be taken at a separate time from zinc during the day.
- *Selenium*: 200 micrograms (mcg). Selenium is toxic in higher doses.
- *Chromium*: 200–300 mcg. Chromium picolinate may help lose weight, and may help lower the necessary dose of niacin.
- *L-taurine*: 500–2,000 mg between meals.
- *L-cysteine*: 500–2,200 mg between meals.
- *L-carnitine*: 500–1,500 mg between meals.
- *Co-Q-10*: 30 mg 1–3 times per day.
- *Pantetheine*: 100–1,200 mg.
- *Omega-3 fatty acids*: 1,000–10,000 mg (with 150–1,500 EPA, the active fatty acid).
- *Chondroitin sulfate*: It has not been established how well chondroitin sulfate is absorbed; doses usually prescribed range from 25 to 100 mg.

In the next chapter, you'll learn about the second of our three "first-tier" strategies for fighting heart disease: increased physical activity. Indeed, in January, 1993, the American Heart Association officially proclaimed inactivity one of the top three risk factors for heart attack and stroke, just after cigarette smoking and high cholesterol levels. The prescription for *everyone*, then, is exercise.

"He lives

most life

whoever breathes

most air."

Elizabeth Barrett Browning

6

Exercising for a Healthy Heart

To the human body, oxygen is energy and life. In fact, the food we eat would be useless without oxygen to break it down so that it becomes available to every cell in our body as energy. Simply stated, without oxygen, cells die and organs cease to function. All it takes is four minutes without oxygen and the brain becomes irreversibly damaged. If heart tissue is denied oxygen, a heart attack results.

In many Eastern philosophies, including Ayurvedic and Chinese medicine, the breath is more than a way to physically sustain the life force of cells. It is also the vehicle of the original cosmic energy that has brought everything else into being. According to these traditions, how much air we take in controls how energy affects the health of the body and mind, as we'll explore in later chapters. In this chapter, we'll be focusing specifically on how increasing our intake of oxygen through physical exercise can improve the health of our cardiovascular system and thus prevent or reverse heart disease.

On the average, we breathe about 20,000 times every day. With every breath we take, trillions of oxygen molecules enter our lungs and seep into the bloodstream through tiny air sacs called alveoli. Once inside the blood, oxygen binds with hemoglobin, the iron-rich part of the red blood cell. The blood is then pumped on to tissues throughout the body. Once oxygen reaches the cells, it is combined with blood sugar, or glucose, to cause tiny combustion reactions within the cells; these reactions release the energy the cells need to function.

The amount of air you breathe depends upon the oxygen demands of your body. During sedentary periods, the average adult takes about 10 to 14 breaths per minute, receiving about 9 to 12 pints of air. During vigorous and sustained exercise, on the other hand, that same adult breathes about twice as fast and much more deeply, increasing intake to approximately 20 gallons of air per minute.

Taking In More Vital Oxygen

You breathe more when you exercise because your muscles signal your brain that they need more energy—and thus more oxygen—to perform their work. In turn, the brain signals the heart to pump harder and the blood pressure to rise (temporarily) so that more oxygen-rich blood is delivered to the muscles and other tissues.

Exercise is often perceived as a painful, tedious process, especially by those who need it most. Properly performed, however, regular exercise soon becomes a positive, life-enhancing habit. Increased physical activity is associated with longer life, and can dramatically improve the quality of life in the old and young alike. It allows you to connect with your physical body in an intimate way, feeling your muscles grow stronger, your heart beat harder, the tension of the day slipping away. To many people, exercise is a time for the intellect to take a back seat to the physical body. Indeed, exercise provides a positive foundation for a generally healthier, more satisfying daily existence for all who partake.

The purely physical benefits of exercise are numerous: Your heart will be able to pump more blood and your vessels will be able to deliver more oxygen to the cells throughout the body in a more efficient manner. Over time, blood cholesterol levels are reduced and the ratio of HDLs (the good cholesterol) to LDLs (the bad cholesterol) is increased. This will help reduce atherosclerosis, one of the major risk factors of heart attack and stroke. Over the long haul, exercise has been shown to reduce blood pressure, as well as increase blood flow into the smallest arteries and veins, thus ensuring that every cell in the body receives proper nutrition.

The heart itself also benefits from a good workout: Because your muscles need more oxygen when they're at work, the heart must pump harder to get extra oxygen-rich blood to them. Normally, the heart pumps about 6 quarts of blood a minute in an average adult man, but when the body is exercising, blood volume to and from the heart rises to about 25 quarts per minute. This extra work strengthens the heart muscle; the stronger it is, the less hard it has to work to meet the body's need for oxygen.

In addition, exercise has significant psychological and emotional benefits. People who exercise find they not only feel better physically, but also have a renewed sense of emotional well-being both during and in-between exercise sessions. Individuals who learn to make exercise a habit in their lives also often increase their self-esteem by setting and reaching new exercise goals.

Part of the reason exercise feels so good is that certain body chemicals called endorphins, known to dull pain and invoke mild euphoria, are released whenever the body feels pain, including the mild discomfort created during vigorous workouts when the muscles begin to tire and "burn." Produced in the spinal cord and the brain, endorphins serve as a perfect example of the body's power to return itself to a state of balance and may be the reason that exercise appears to reduce anxiety and stress in those who undertake it on a regular basis. Smokers who exercise find it easier to quit. Therapists frequently prescribe exercise to their depressed patients. And dieters who exercise claim to feel less hungry and more self-confident about meeting their weight loss goals than they did when they were sedentary.

It is important to note that exercise need not be demanding or elaborate to be effective: A recent study at the USDA Human Nutrition Research Center on Aging at Tufts University showed that nonathletes who merely moved around a lot in their daily lives had less body fat than those who were more sedentary.

That means that simply by adding a few vigorous daily chores—like gardening with extra energy, performing strenuous housework, even taking the stairs instead of the elevator at work on a regular basis—will take you a long way on the journey toward cardiovascular health. A study published in the *Journal of the American Medical Association* in November, 1989, showed that moderate exercise—defined as 30 minutes a day of light activity such as walking and gardening—is almost as beneficial to one's health as higher levels of exercise, such as high-impact aerobics and jogging. Moreover, moderate exercise is far safer than high-intensity activities for those people who have already been diagnosed with heart disease or who have been sedentary in recent months or years.

Exercises for a Healthy Heart

In essence, there are two basic types of exercise: aerobic and anaerobic. The purpose of aerobic exercise is to improve cardiovascular health by forcing the body to deliver ever larger amounts of oxygen to working muscles. In fact, the word aerobic is derived from a Greek word meaning "air."

Anaerobic exercise (exercise "without air"), on the other hand, attempts to strengthen individual muscles. Because such exertion requires more oxygen, quickly, than breathing can supply, the muscles draw on their own sources of energy, stored in the tissues, and do not require the body to increase its supply of oxygen. Also known as muscle conditioning or weight training, anaerobic exercise tries to build muscle mass and keep the body strong and flexible.

In addition to discussing these two basic types of exercise, this chapter will also explore the physical benefits of yoga, a system of exercise and meditation developed largely in India. Some yoga postures work directly to increase circulation, helping to strengthen blood vessels and heart tissue; those postures will be illustrated in this chapter. Depending on the speed and intensity with which the exercises are performed, yoga can be either aerobic or anaerobic. (In Chapter 7, you'll discover the spiritual and meditative qualities of yoga as they relate to relaxation and stress reduction.)

Generally speaking, aerobic exercise is considered the most beneficial to the cardiovascular system because it increases the amount of oxygen the body receives. Indeed, the effects of aerobics, which uses large muscle groups to get the heart pumping and the lungs filling with oxygen, are substantial. With aerobic exercise, your body learns to burn fat more efficiently for fuel, a definite boon for people trying to lose excess weight to reduce the burden of extra weight on their cardiovascular system.

New studies indicate that combining aerobics with some weight-training (anaerobic exercise) may be the best way to achieve overall health and fitness—especially if you are overweight. Muscle is more metabolically active than fat: which simply means that the body must burn more calories to feed and nourish muscle tissue than it would to maintain fat. Therefore, the more muscle you have, the more calories you'll burn every day.

In addition to cardiovascular and muscle conditioning, many people are adding another, often overlooked, component of a healthy exercise plan: flexibility. Good flexibility is thought to protect the muscles against pulls and tears; short, tight muscles may be more likely to be overstretched. Yoga exercises, which stretch muscles slowly and steadily while bathing the cells in oxygen through deep breathing, are particularly effective in promoting flexibility and increased circulation.

AEROBIC EXERCISE

Aerobic exercise generally involves working large muscle groups, such as leg muscles, for a sustained length of time, generally more than 20 minutes at a steady, moderate pace. Included among the best aerobic exercises are walking, jogging, aerobic dance, stair-climbing and step classes, cross-country skiing, rowing, and vigorous cycling. As we'll discuss below, walking at a strong and steady pace is the easiest, safest, and healthiest way to get your heart pumping and your body burning more energy.

No matter what type of aerobic exercise you choose, you'll want to satisfy three basic criteria: *intensity*, *duration*, and *frequency*. It is important to note that these are optimal goals: You should not expect to achieve all three the first week you begin to exercise. The key to safe and effective exercise is to start slowly and build gradually. Now let's take the criteria for aerobic exercise one by one:

First, in order for exercise to have the maximum effect on the cardiovascular system, aerobic exercise should be of a sufficient *intensity*. You should exercise at a level of intensity called your target heart rate, or the rate at which your heart must work to provide health benefits to the cardiovascular system. At this rate, you will burn about 300 calories in 30 minutes.

Target heart rates are calculated by using a simple formula. Your target heart rate is between 70 and 85 percent of your maximum heart rate; your maximum heart rate is calculated by subtracting your age from 220. For the average 30-year-old, then, the maximum heart rate would be 220–30, or 190; the target heart range should be from 133 to 162 beats per minute, or 70 to 85 percent of the maximum heart rate.

You can determine whether or not you are within your target zone by taking your pulse immediately after exercise. Some exercisers choose to monitor their pulses periodically during the session. The easiest way to take your pulse is to place two fingers (not your thumb, as it is also a pulse point and can disturb the accuracy of your reading) on your wrist. Count the beats for 10 seconds, then multiply that number by 6. If your pulse rate is below the target range, you should increase either the intensity or the length of your workout. If your pulse is above your target rate, slow down until your pulse falls into the proper range.

In addition to being intense, each aerobic exercise session should have a *duration* of about 20 to 30 minutes, especially if you're trying to lose weight. When you first start to exercise, your muscles draw on quick sources of energy within their own cells, which can be obtained without increasing the body's supply of oxygen. The longer you exercise, though, the more oxygen you'll need, the harder your heart will pump, and the more your body draws on stored fat as energy. Again, don't worry if you are not able to exercise for 30 minutes right away; take it slow and build gradually.

Finally, to achieve lasting cardiovascular benefits, you must exercise on a *regular* basis. You should aim for exercising about three to five days per week, preferably at your target heart rate for about half an hour. Don't get discouraged if you are not able to meet that schedule at first: Every time you move your body, you're doing something positive for your health, even if it's just for 10 extra minutes a day.

EXERCISE TIP

Time your exercise carefully, especially if you live in the city where the air is likely to be especially polluted with potentially harmful toxins like carbon monoxide, sulfur dioxide, and ozone. Athough studies have not yet made clear whether repeated exposure to pollutants during exercise can result in disease or lung damage, it would seem wise to avoid exercising near moderately heavy traffic or during the early afternoon when ozone levels tend to be highest. If you are unable to fit your outdoor walk or jog into optimally healthy times, you might want to consider joining a gym and exercising indoors.

On the other hand, to really experience a difference in the way you feel about your body and your health, you'll need to make exercise a regular part of your life.

That's why it is crucial for you to choose an activity you enjoy. Think of it this way: If you exercise three times a week for 30 minutes a session, at the end of a year's time, you'll have stair-stepped, jogged, or rowed for about 78 hours—the equivalent of two solid workweeks. If you're like an increasing number of Americans, you'll think about choosing one of the most effective, safest, and enjoyable aerobic activities known to man or woman: Walking.

WALKING YOUR WAY TOWARD HEALTH

Did you know that walking a mile burns only about 15 percent fewer calories than jogging a mile? That even walking at a slow pace will burn 80 calories per hour? Injuries are minimized by walking instead of jogging or running, walking can be done at any time of the day and anywhere in the world, and the natural rhythm of walking can foster the meditative qualities of exercise.

If you decide to take up walking as part of your exercise routine, follow these simple tips:

Start slow. If you're inactive but healthy, start with one-mile walks at a pace of three miles per hour, which means that you should finish a mile in about 20 minutes. Over the course of a month, gradually increase your distance to three miles at a pace of about four miles per hour (about 15 minutes per mile). Try to schedule walks from three to five times per week.

Wear proper footwear. Although there is no need for you to spend lots of money on fancy walking shoes or sneakers, you should choose a shoe that has a rigid arch and some cushioning on the heel and ball of the foot. Such support will help keep your body properly aligned as you walk.

Vary your route and your routine. If possible, take the time to map out two or three different routes to avoid becoming bored by taking the same walk every day. As you become more physically fit, head for the hills. You'll burn more calories and your heart will work even harder when you walk up an incline. Even walking downhill requires about four times as much effort as walking on a level surface.

Use your arms as well as your legs. Once you feel comfortable walking at a pace of about 3½ miles per hour, you might be ready to increase the aerobic benefits of your workout by adding an upper body component. Swinging your arms vigorously in pace with your steps will help increase your heart rate, as will wearing light (one-pound) arm or hand weights.

Contemplate your environment. Walking provides you with the time and personal space in which to observe your surroundings and appreciate nature. Perhaps for the first time since childhood, you'll be able to take note of the trees and flowers in the park, the architecture of the buildings lining the city streets, the quality of the fresh air as it passes through your nostrils and mouth. Time your walks to coincide with sunrise or sunset, watch the seasons change as you feel yourself getting stronger, healthier, and more relaxed.

ANAEROBIC EXERCISE

Anaerobic exercises, including calisthenics and weight training (with free weights or with Nautilus), are not usually recommended for people with high blood pressure or advanced cardiovascular disease of any type. Such exercises may cause temporary but marked rises in blood pressure; unless you receive permission from your physician or alternate practitioner, you should stick with increasing your cardio-vascular capabilities with aerobic exercise.

On the other hand, if you have normal blood pressure and are in relatively good health, adding strength training to your exercise routine may be both helpful and enjoyable. It takes more energy for your body to nourish muscle tissue than to maintain fat. So the more muscular you are, the more fat you'll burn and the easier it will be for you to lose weight if you need to.

Because the techniques of calisthenics and weight training are very precise and, if not performed properly, can lead to injury, we suggest that you visit a local gym or YMCA to receive firsthand instruction before you try to begin a program on your own. A **weight-training** routine should involve about 30 minutes of steady—but constant—stress on different muscles of the body using your own body weight (calisthenics), free weights, or strength-training equipment (such as Nautilus). Your exact exercise routine should be formulated with an exercise specialist in a gym, but generally speaking it consists of about a dozen exercises: six for the upper body and six for the lower.

EXERCISE TIP

"No pain, no gain" is a myth, and a dangerous one at that. Exercise should require some effort, but actual pain is a warning sign that your muscles are being strained beyond what is healthy. If you experience continuing pain during an exercise, stop immediately and do not repeat the exercise until you can do so without feeling pain.

STRETCHING AND YOGA POSTURES

Most Americans, even those who consider themselves to be in top physical condition, neglect flexibility. Part of the reason may lie in the noncompetitive nature of stretching; unlike aerobics and weight training, there are no times or weight limits to beat. Instead, stretching the muscles slowly and steadily to their limit and slightly beyond is an intensely personal effort, one that brings an individual closer to truly understanding the unique structure of his or her own body.

Every exercise session should begin with a short aerobic warm-up (like jogging in place) and then a series of movements designed to stretch the muscles you'll be working during your aerobic and/or weight-training phase. If you'll be playing tennis or walking, for instance, you'll want to stretch your calf muscles and the muscles in the upper back and shoulders. Here are some of the most common stretching exercises:

Shoulders/upper back. Raise your right arm and reach down your back as far as you can. At the same time, place your left arm behind your back and try to reach the fingers of your right hand. Sustain this stretch for 5 to 10 seconds. Repeat with arms reversed.

Chest/arms. Stand sideways and at arm's length from a wall. Reach out and slightly behind you and place one palm on the wall. Keep your hand in place, turn your body away slightly. Hold the stretch for 5 to 10 seconds. Repeat with the other arm.

Calves. Lean forward on the balls of your feet, heels lifted, and bounce, very gently 20 times. Then, at slightly less than arm's length and with heels on the floor, lean toward a wall, supporting your weight on both hands. Keep your legs straight and heels on the ground. Hold the stretch for 10 seconds.

Hamstrings. (The hamstrings are the large muscles at the backs of your thighs.) Place one foot about 12 inches in front of the other. Raise the toes of the leading foot in the air. Keeping both knees slightly bent, lean your torso forward as if you were taking a bow. Feel the stretch, for about 10 seconds, in the back and front of your thigh. Reverse the position.

Quite apart from stretching before other exercise, however, there is another system of movement that increases circulation and flexibility in a systematic and often intense way. The system, known as yoga, has been practiced for centuries in the East and, especially since the early twentieth century, in the West as well. As you'll discover in Chapters 7 and 10, meditation and proper breathing techniques are essential components of a comprehensive yoga program. However, there are a few yoga exercises that promote cardiovascular health which can be added to your daily stretching routine.

The specific postures helpful in increasing circulation and releasing energy to the heart and blood vessels are as follows:

Chest expansion posture. Hold your arms out at the sides, and slowly move them backward until you can interlace your hands behind your body, at about shoulder level. (You'll have to bend your elbows.) Slowly stretch your arms up without straining, holding your trunk straight. Then stretch the arms backward and gently arch your back, holding the stretch for about 5 seconds. Then slowly bend your body forward, dropping your head and raising your arms behind your head, for about 10 seconds. Finally, drop arms to your sides and relax.

Cobra posture. Lie face down, with your hands under your shoulders facing each other. Begin raising your head and lifting your chest by pushing with your hands. When your arms are straight, your head should be held up and your back should be gently arched for a count of 10 seconds. Then reverse the motions until you're lying relaxed on the floor. Repeat.

Shoulder stand posture. Lying on the floor facing up, slowly raise your legs upward, allowing your hips to rise off the floor until your head and shoulders are supporting the rest of the body. If this is difficult, the posture can be done against a wall to support your hips and legs. Hold your legs up in the air for 30 seconds or more, then lower them and relax.

Creating an Exercise Plan

With or without a diagnosis of cardiovascular disease, your first step in starting an exercise program is to consult with your physician and/or alternative practitioner, especially if you're overweight, over 40, or have any other risk factors for cardiovascular disease.

Your health practitioner may recommend that you take a stress test, which measures how your heart and blood vessels are functioning. A stress test involves nothing more than having your heart rate measured by an ECG (electrocardiogram) and your blood pressure monitored by a technician while you jog on a treadmill or ride a stationary bicycle. One of the most important benefits of the stress test is that it helps diagnose heart and vessel disease. It will also help determine the amount of exercise your heart and muscles can handle without any adverse effects. Knowing both the length of time you are able to exercise and the intensity of activity you are able to endure without becoming exhausted will help your doctor determine a safe exercise routine for you.

What kind of exercise or exercises should you perform? In general, if you're concerned about cardiovascular disease, you should start by increasing your aerobic activity. Aerobic exercise is the most efficient way to build cardiovascular endurance and reduce the risks or reverse the damage of heart disease. You can decide to walk, take an aerobics class, use a rowing machine, or alternate these activities. If you would like to add other elements, such as weight training and/or yoga, you can build that into your program simultaneously or after you become accustomed to exercising aerobically on a regular basis.

Regardless of the type of exercise you choose, every session should contain three elements: (1) a warm-up, (2) a cardiovascular phase, and (3) a cool-down. Ideally, the entire session should last about 45 minutes.

1. A 5- to 10-minute *warm-up* is essential before any physical exercise, aerobic or anaerobic. Warming up prepares you for exercise by gradually increasing your heart rate, blood flow, and muscle action. Contrary to popular belief, however, a good warm-up does not begin with stretching; stretching cold muscles can injure them. Instead, you should jog in place for a minute or two before you start to stretch. When you do stretch, it's best to gently work the muscles you are planning to use (your legs if you are walking or running, for instance).

2. The *aerobic phase* of the exercise should last approximately 30 minutes at your target heart rate to give you the most benefit. However, beginners who are out of shape may have trouble sustaining intense exercise for that long. Many experts suggest reducing this phase of the workout session to about 5 to 10 minutes for a few weeks until your heart and muscles have gained some capacity and strength.

It is important that if you feel any of the following symptoms while exercising, *stop exercising immediately and consult your physician to determine the basis of the symptoms.* They could be signs of some cardiovascular stress, such as a heart attack or stroke:

- Chest discomfort, including pain, tightness, heaviness, or breathlessness

- Any discomfort or numbness in the jaw, neck, or arm
- Dizziness
- Headache
- Nausea

If you decide you would like to strengthen your muscles as well as work your cardiovascular system—and if you've received permission from your physician—a *weight-training* and muscle-conditioning routine could either come after an aerobic workout (but before the cooldown) or be performed on a separate day, after an appropriate warm-up.

3. The third phase of your workout session is called the *cooldown*. It consists of two parts. First, gradually reduce the intensity level of whatever activity you're performing. If you choose to jog, for instance, don't suddenly stop and sit down. Instead, walk a block or two at a somewhat slower pace. Cooling down will both help you avoid muscle stiffness and reduce the chances of an abrupt drop in blood pressure that can occur when exercise comes to a sudden halt. Then stretch gently for about five minutes. At this time, you may choose to perform the yoga postures described above.

KEYS TO MAINTAINING YOUR EXERCISE PROGRAM

You've checked with your doctor. You've started to exercise, and you've been keeping to a pretty regular schedule of three workouts per week. You know in your heart that your exercise program should last forever, that regular exercise must become a part of your daily life if lasting health benefits are to be derived. But you've seen others fail in their same very good intentions. Perhaps you've failed before, too.

To help you stick to an exercise routine, try one or more of these hints:

Choose activities you enjoy. Perhaps the most important element in the design of your exercise program is choosing activities you will enjoy over the long haul. Very often people start exercising with great enthusiasm, but after just a few weeks revert to their former sedentary ways. Boredom, inconvenience, and lack of motivation are all at the top of former exercisers' reasons for quitting.

Start slowly. Don't overdo your exercising in the first few days. If you do, you are likely to become sore and discouraged, perhaps even ready to discontinue your workout plan. The best way to stick to exercising is to start small and build gradually.

Set realistic goals. If you've been sedentary for a number of months or years, deciding to train for next month's marathon by running 10 miles every morning would be counterproductive and even dangerous to your health. After failing to meet the unrealistic goal, or straining your muscles trying to do so, you'd become frustrated and probably decide not to exercise at all. Instead, set goals you know you can meet, or perhaps ones just out of reach. Achieving them will give you a sense of pride and self-confidence sure to keep you motivated.

Add variety. To alleviate boredom, you may want to alternate activities, taking a dance class one session, bicycling outside for 45 minutes the next, performing yoga postures every other morning. By varying your routine, you're more likely to keep it going.

Seek convenience. Another hint to help you stick to an exercise program is to eliminate as many excuses as possible for not exercising. If you join a health club that is only open during hours you are at work, for instance, then obviously you're setting yourself up to fail. Scheduling times to exercise—and treating your exercise times as if they were business appointments—is often the only way to incorporate aerobic activity into your lifestyle.

Find a support group. For most of us, there comes a time when our motivation sags and we lose interest in exercising on a regular basis. When this happens—preferably *before* this happens—enlist a friend or loved one to join you in your quest for cardiovascular health. Often, a little friendly competition and companionship go a long way.

Regular exercise has one special benefit especially important to those suffering from cardiovascular disease: It serves as a great method of reducing stress. In Chapter 7, we'll describe other techniques for relieving the emotional pressures that may be preventing you from achieving a more balanced state of mind and body, a state known as health.

"Anger or revolt that does not get into the muscles remains a figment of the imagination."

Simone de Beauvoir

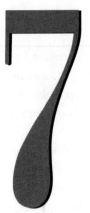

Stress Reduction
and Relaxation

At the young age of 36, Melinda Douglas underwent a triple bypass operation, an open-heart surgical procedure deemed necessary because all three of Melinda's coronary arteries were blocked by atherosclerosis. Blood flow to her heart was severely restricted and she was at high risk for a heart attack in the near future. Following the operation, Melinda was prescribed medication to reduce her blood pressure by dilating the peripheral blood vessels. Her doctor felt she was depressed, and began an antidepressant as well.

Within just a few months, however, Melinda began to experience chest pains once again. Because the surgery and recovery period had been unpleasant, Melinda decided to seek alternative therapy for her condition and came to me for help. In particular, she sought relief from her chest pains, explaining to me that "They seem to come whenever I get upset or anxious, which is often."

On examination, I found Melinda to have extremely tense muscles in her upper back, neck, and chest areas. She did not move her chest a lot when she inhaled and was unable to freely move her neck from side to side. She also constantly had the look of someone who had just been startled.

I talked with her about her health and her life in general for about an hour. During the course of our conversation, I found out that Melinda had been struggling for years with intimacy issues; she had been through two failed marriages and was currently feeling very lonely. She felt generally unsatisfied with her job as a waitress, which she also found to be quite stressful.

After hearing her story and examining her, I discussed with Melinda the way in which her tight muscles and breathing mechanism were attempting to "guard" her heart from the hurt she felt would come with intimacy. Instead of protecting her from harm, however, her muscular tension was adding to her cardiovascular problems by keeping her blood from circulating freely. I held out the possibility that by opening this area by deep breathing and muscle relaxation, she could increase the blood flow to her heart area and thus reduce her angina.

I presented the many stress reduction and breathing techniques to Melinda. She decided to try working first with biofeedback, learning to relax her upper back and chest muscles, to increase the blood flow to her hands, and to breathe deeply into her abdominal area. As she developed a better sense of relaxation, some of her emotions began to surface, particularly her sadness over her isolation from others and her frustration about her job. Melinda decided to seek help from a psychotherapist to work through some of these issues more comprehensively.

Working with her therapist and with me as her biofeedback "coach," Melinda learned some useful techniques to relax, breathe deeply, and increase her circulation, both in general and during particularly anxious or tense situations. Three months after beginning this work, Melinda was free of angina and off of her antidepressant medicine.

Stress, a Heart Poison

High blood pressure, high cholesterol and lipid levels, poor glucose metabolism—all of these risk factors for heart disease can be identified and measured by scientifically accepted methods. For that reason, mainstream medicine has concentrated on assessing and treating these medical problems during much of the twentieth century, for the most part leaving aside another integral part of the cardiovascular picture: the effect of stress on the heart, blood, and blood vessels.

The difficulty many physicians have in assessing stress is three-fold: First, except for extreme situations, like the death of a loved one or the threat of imminent physical harm, a clear definition of stress is not available. Everything that occurs in your life or exists in the atmosphere is technically a stressor because it affects you in some way. If it is very hot out, for instance, your body will adjust to the increased temperature by cooling the skin with perspiration. In this instance, heat is a stressor because it spurs the body to action. If you receive an unexpected bonus from your boss, the excitement the event stimulates may make your heart beat faster, your muscles tense up, your palms sweat. Despite its positive impact, then, the news of your bonus is a stressor because it forces a physiological reaction—one that will be described in more depth below—to occur.

A second problem in relating stress to disease involves how variable our reactions to stress tend to be. Clearly, not everyone responds to stress in the same way. Some people become outwardly aggravated over the slightest mishap while others never blink an eye even when disaster occurs. It should be noted, however, that the outwardly calm person may be actually seething inside, perhaps negatively affecting his or her physiology even more than the person who expresses anger and frustration in a more open way.

Third, and even more significantly, stressors vary from person to person. For some, a day spent lying on a beach is completely relaxing, while for others such forced recreation is sheer (often blood-pressure-raising) torture. It is how you as an individual perceive an event that determines how your body reacts to it.

Despite the difficulties in defining and measuring stress, it has become increasingly clear to even the most hard-nosed mainstream physicians that a connection exists between the mind, the emotions, and health. In the study of heart disease, in particular, evidence has begun to mount that excess stress increases the amount of cholesterol in the blood, thus contributing to the development of atherosclerosis. Stress may also increase the heart rate and raise blood pressure. In many individuals, including Melinda, stress results in decreased circulation to the heart muscle itself, often causing the pain known as angina.

Fortunately, it is possible to learn to control both the way you perceive stress and how your body copes with it, at least to a certain extent. Before we discuss relaxation methods with you, however, it is important that you gain an understanding of how stress affects your cardiovascular system and how you, as an individual, may be affected by stress.

The Physiology of Stress

If you've ever doubted that there is a connection between your emotions and your internal physiology, just think about the first time you fell in love. When you looked across the room and saw the object of your affection, didn't your heart beat faster? Didn't your palms sweat? Didn't you feel as if you might faint because the blood had rushed from your head to your feet as you tried to make your way to the one you loved?

In addition to infatuation, what you were feeling was fear and anticipation—of rejection, of commitment, of the unknown, perhaps even of success—and your body sensed your emotions. In a completely instinctive and interdependent way, your brain, your hormones, and your nervous system worked to prepare you to face what you perceived as a threat to your emotional, if not physical, safety.

Whether you are conscious of it or not, your body has a remarkable gift for self-preservation. When its internal balance is threatened in any way, it mobilizes immediately, preparing you either to battle the impending danger or to flee from it. We're perhaps more used to thinking of this response, known as the "fight-or-flight response," as occurring during times of physical danger: Out of nowhere, it seems, a bus bears down on you while you're crossing the street. Your heart starts to pound and the muscles in your legs and arms tense up. Before you know it, you're safely across the street, running faster and harder than you'd thought possible.

The sight of your new love and the sight of the bus set off the same chain of reactions in your body. As soon as a threat to your internal harmony is perceived—positive or negative—your body goes into action. In fact, it is no longer possible to discuss a separation between what we think and feel and our physical selves; they are one and the same. You see a bus coming toward you and your heart starts to pound. Thinking back, you recall you felt afraid, and one of the physical manifestations of that fear was your heart beating faster and stronger. You've been taught by mainstream medicine to think that your brain "told" your heart to beat faster and your muscles to tense up. However, recent research is showing that your mind exists not only in your brain, but in cells and tissues throughout your body.

In particular, two interrelated systems, the autonomic nervous system and the endocrine system, become more active during times of stress. These two systems are so directly related to what is occurring to us emotionally and intellectually that they can be considered the physical representatives of emotions within the body.

The autonomic nervous system controls bodily functions like the heartbeat, intestinal movements, salivation, and other activities of the internal organs. It is divided into two parts that work to balance these activities: The sympathetic nervous system speeds up heart rate, narrows blood vessels, and raises blood pressure during times of physical or emotional stress, while the parasympathetic nervous system works to slow these processes down when the body perceives that the stress has passed.

Indeed, the two parts of the autonomic system represent a perfect example of the balance we know of as health. In Chinese medicine, the sympathetic nervous system is the "yang" and the parasympathetic system is the "yin" of the body and its responses. Bringing your body into harmony during and after stressful periods, by triggering your parasympathetic nervous system into action, is as important to your health as is reacting immediately, through the sympathetic nervous system, to the perceived threats known as stressors.

Directly related to nervous system activity are hormones secreted by the glands of the endocrine system. The glands release stress hormones into the bloodstream that, in turn, produce various reactions in the organs and tissues of the body. These hormones are norepinephrine and epinephrine (also called adrenaline). These two hormones are known as catecholamines. Secreted by the adrenal medulla (the internal part of the adrenal gland) and the sympathetic nerve endings themselves, catecholamines stimulate the sympathetic nervous system to raise the blood pressure, continue to increase the heart rate, increase the metabolic rate, and make you breathe faster to provide more oxygen to your muscles. They also increase platelet stickiness, increase the possibility of dangerous arrhythmias and strokes, and cause spasm of coronary arteries.

The autonomic nervous system and catecholimines work together, electrically and biochemically, to provide a fast and usually short-lived response to an immediate threat. Other hormones allow the body to continue fighting long after the effects of the fight-or-flight response are over. From the surface of the adrenal gland, called the adrenal cortex, come two types of steroid hormones known as glucocorticoids and mineralocorticoids. The primary glucocorticoid is the hormone cortisol and the primary mineralocorticoid is aldosterone. During times of acute stress, both of these hormones provide fuel for battle.

Cortisol works primarily to increase the blood sugar so that we have energy for action. In addition, cortisol pulls fatty acids from fat tissue and breaks down protein, to provide quick extra energy. It also suppresses inflammation. Aldosterone, on the other hand, increases blood pressure so that we can transport food and oxygen to the active parts of our body; it does so by decreasing urine production and increasing sodium retention, both of which will increase the blood volume and thus the pressure at which blood travels through the body.

As you can see, the body works hard to keep you safe from acute danger. However, problems occur when these powerful hormones and the reactions they stimulate continue over a long period of time. So it's *chronic* stress that causes illness in most cases. Here are just a few of the ways chronic stress affects the cardiovascular system in a negative way:

- Blood pressure remains elevated and the heart beats harder and faster than it should.
- Excess cortisol may also lead to elevated blood sugar, platelet stickiness, and, some research shows, an increased level of serum cholesterol in the blood.
- Norepinephrine and epinephrine are able to injure arterial walls, further paving the way for atherosclerosis.
- All of the stress hormones have a tendency to increase free radical formation. Free radicals are dangerous molecules that may lead to the oxidation of cholesterol. And oxidized cholesterol is the "bad" cholesterol that damages blood vessels and may lead to heart disease.
- Chronic muscle tension can deplete the body's store of magnesium and potassium, creating an excess of calcium and sodium. These two latter minerals may act to cause vasospasm—abnormal constriction of the arteries, including the coronary arteries which may result in a heart attack. Some studies have shown that about 50 percent of heart attacks may be caused by coronary spasm alone, not by blockage of the coronary arteries by atherosclerosis.

Simply put, chronic stress provides your body with all the ingredients necessary for serious cardiovascular disease. How and why does chronic stress occur? In today's fast-paced society, it often seems as if we don't have time to recover from one stressful situation before getting hit by another. You survive nearly being hit by a bus only to reach the office to find that one of your clients needs a file immedi-ately. You head for the photocopier, only to find that it's broken. Attempting to fix it, you stab your hand with an errant piece of machinery . . . and you know how the rest of the day is bound to go.

In addition, the more stress you feel, the more likely you are to engage in other high-risk behaviors, like smoking and drinking too much, overeating, and exercising too little. Although you may feel that these habits help to relax you, they are, in fact, increasing the stress on your body by forcing it to cope with the ill effects of these substances and behaviors. Because your body is constantly struggling to keep itself in the state of internal balance we know of as health, the more physical and emotional stress you must deal with, the more difficult it is for your health to be maintained.

Since our world is so filled with stress-producing events and environmental toxins, shouldn't everyone suffer from cardiovascular disease? Although cardiovascular disease is the most common chronic condition in the Western world, it is true that not everyone is affected equally by stress, either emotionally or physically. Next, we'll discuss what may make one individual more prone to stress-related disease than another.

Test Your Coping Behavior

It is important for you to gain an understanding of how stress may be affecting your behavior. Check off the statements that apply to the way you behave in your daily life.

1. ___ I move and speak rapidly.
2. ___ I feel impatient with the rate at which most events take place.
3. ___ I hurry the speech of others, often finishing their sentences.
4. ___ I find it difficult to wait in line.
5. ___ I find it intolerable to watch others perform tasks I know I can do faster.
6. ___ I frequently strive to think about or do two or more things simultaneously.

7. ___   I feel guilty when not working or performing
         useful chores.
8. ___   I attempt to schedule more and more in less and
         less time.
9. ___   I feel unworthy of any success I've achieved.
10. ___ I feel lonely and isolated.

How many of the statements applied to the way you behave in your daily life? If you found yourself relating to more than one or two of them, you may be what has been termed as a "Type A" personality and thus at special risk for stress-related cardiovascular disease.

Scientists have determined that it is not only the *amount* of stress we face but also how we cope with stress that affects our health. Our understanding of how personality relates to cardiovascular disease was fostered by two California cardiologists, Drs. Meyer Friedman and Ray Rosenman in the mid-1970s. By studying the behavior of their fellow doctors and their patients, Drs. Friedman and Rosenman discovered that people with heart disease were more likely to display certain behaviors than their healthy counterparts.

Specifically, heart disease was more common in people they termed "Type A"; these people tended to be more demanding, ambitious, and hostile. They hurried conversations, focused almost exclusively on themselves, tried to perform more than one task at a time, and frequently overscheduled their days and nights with activities. Success for a typical Type A personality was based on quantifiable measurements: the highest grade in school, the largest salary, sales figures, etc. Unable to relax—and feeling guilty when they attempted to do so—Type A's displayed many physical signs of stress as well, including clenching of the fists and jaws, wringing of the hands, or, like Melinda in the case study above, muscular tension in the shoulders, back, and neck.

Those with less evidence of heart disease, termed Type B, were more calm and easygoing. Although equally ambitious and successful in many cases, Type B personalities were more open and patient with others and more interested in what others felt and had to say. Type Bs took time out each day to relax, and felt little or no guilt in doing so. In essence, Type B personalities are able to balance stress with relaxation, while Type A personalities exist in a state of mental, and thus physical, tension.

In a study conducted at Duke University in North Carolina, this theory was put to a test. More than 3,000 mostly white men—1,500 Type As and 1,500 Type Bs—were followed to see the effect their personalities had on their health. After eight years, it was found that Type A men had significantly more atherosclerosis than Type B men. It was calculated that the increase in atherosclerosis put the Type A men at twice the risk of the Type B men for having a heart attack.

Since Drs. Friedman and Rosenman's groundbreaking study, further research on behavior and its relationship to heart disease has been done. The evidence is strong that people whose lives or jobs make high demands on them but allow little latitude for decision-making have higher rates of many diseases. Although we think of the Type A personality as having "executive stress," it's the people at the *other* end of the ladder who are more likely to suffer from stress and its ill effects. Those in high-strain, low-echelon jobs are more likely than executives, who have more freedom in their jobs, to suffer from stress-related disease. Air-traffic controllers, for instance, are four times as likely to have high blood pressure as pilots; gas station attendants, assembly-line workers, and salespeople in high-pressure fields are more likely to have heart disease than people who have more control over their schedules and productivity.

Other aspects of our psychological makeup are also worth considering in a discussion of stress and heart disease. Self-esteem is an extremely important, and often overlooked, aspect of health. Those who feel that they are destined to fail (and thus have no control over their lives) or that they are unworthy of the success they do achieve tend to feel stress more acutely than others with more confidence in themselves and their ability to alter their environments.

Social isolation may be an even greater indicator of potential health problems than either Type A behavior or a low sense of self-esteem. Living alone, without social support from a church, community, or circle of friends to whom you can express your emotions, appears to significantly increase the risk of heart disease and other illness. One study of heart attack survivors reported in the *New England Journal of Medicine* revealed that people who were classified as being socially isolated had more than four times the risk of death from heart disease compared with those who had low levels of isolation. A ten-year study, which Dr. Dean Ornish cites in his book *Dr. Dean Ornish's Guide to Reversing Heart Disease*, found that social isolation was one of the best predictors of mortality, both from all causes and from coronary heart disease.

More work is needed to help us understand the exact relationship between self-esteem, social isolation, and internal stress, but one thing remains clear: A positive image of ourselves and our lives, and a healthy connection to those around us, are major factors in maintaining good health. Thus keeping an "open heart" becomes not just a phrase, but a prescription.

Fortunately, there are ways to improve the way you cope with the stresses in your life. Your body can learn what is known as the "relaxation response" to counteract the "fight-or-flight response" during times of stress, bringing the body back into balance quickly and efficiently. To do so, you'll be activating your parasympathetic nervous system—your calming yin to counteract your overactive yang—to attain a more peaceful and relaxed internal harmony.

Learning to Relax

Needless to say, one of the most effective ways of reducing the amount of stress you experience is by eliminating as many stress-causing agents from your life as possible: changing your job to one less fraught with tension, moving to a place more suited to your personality and taste, avoiding people who annoy you, etc. Unfortunately, making such changes is easier said than done and will take some long-range planning and, no doubt, a good deal of self-examination.

Indeed, learning what is causing your life to be unbalanced—and what might help you make it more fulfilling—is the first step in the process of gaining control over your health. For some, this may involve confronting serious psychological and social issues, including substance abuse problems, childhood traumas, and other matters that may have eroded self-esteem and self-confidence over the years. For this reason, many people decide to seek the help of a psychologist or psychiatrist in working to resolve some of these issues. Although psychological therapy is certainly not necessary for everyone with heart disease, it is something to consider if you are unsure of how your lifestyle, and life history, may be affecting your health.

In addition, you should take the time now to evaluate your relationships with other people—both your close family and friends and the community at large. As discussed above, social isolation is one of the key predictors of cardiovascular disease and of poor health in general. As you begin to resolve some of your own self-esteem issues, you'll want to at least start the process of opening your heart to others.

Many people find that the best way to do this is to join a support group of some kind, either one directed toward an appropriate health-related issue (like Alcoholics Anonymous or Weight Watchers) or one that focuses on a general subject of interest to you (a church or synagogue, a stamp-collecting club, etc.). You might even be able to kill two birds with one stone: Join a gym or a walking group so that you'll get some exercise while making new friends. (As Chapter 6 pointed out, exercise itself is one of the best stress-relievers available.)

Although making these deeper changes in the way you see yourself and others may be your ultimate stress-reducing goal, there are many physical exercises you can do—starting today—that will result in some significant physical and psychological benefits within a relatively short period of time. All of the methods to be described here—and there are many others—involve bringing your body into a deep state of relaxation by balancing the activities of your sympathetic nervous system with the activities of your parasympathetic nervous system.

Learning to relax your body and your mind will accomplish many health-related goals. It will reduce the time your body remains tense and in the "stress reaction mode" and have a positive effect on your blood pressure, serum cholesterol levels, and your heart rates. You'll learn that you have power and control over your internal environment. Realizing that you can make successful, positive changes in your physical and mental health will automatically raise your self-esteem and give you a new sense of self-confidence. Not only that, coming to terms with your own feelings will help you relate better to others. It will help you "open your heart" both literally and figuratively.

In this chapter, you'll learn about four methods of stress reduction: yogic breathing, progressive relaxation, biofeedback, and meditation. It goes far beyond the scope of this book to cover these subjects, or the many other methods of relaxation available, in the depth that they deserve and it is up to you to continue your research using other books (listed in *An Alternative Medicine Resource Guide*, p. 196) and/or by contacting schools or individual teachers for more guidance.

For now, here's a brief overview of a few effective relaxation strategies.

YOGIC BREATHING

Have you noticed that when you become distressed, your breathing becomes rapid and shallow? When you're more relaxed, on the other hand, you're probably breathing more slowly and regularly and your breath may be coming from your stomach area rather than your chest. When you are tired, have you noticed that taking a deep breath makes you more alert? Or when you're attempting to concentrate, that breathing in helps you to improve your performance?

In fact, your breath, or more accurately your breathing process, forms a link between your sympathetic and parasympathetic nervous systems. By learning to breathe deeply and regularly, you can help foster a healthy balance between your internal yin and yang. Many Eastern philosophies look at the breath as being far more than mere oxygen. The breath is cosmic energy; it operates in the working of all of our body processes and is at the same time the universal life-force in which we all share. Air is energy, and, by using proper breathing techniques, we can learn how to tap that energy source to help bring our bodies into balance.

Yoga, a system of exercises developed in India and Tibet, focuses on using the breath to provide energy and relaxation. There are several different forms of yogic breathing. Some are meant to cleanse the body of impurities, others to help guide us toward spiritual enlightenment. For our immediate purposes we'll focus on a relatively easy and very effective exercise called "The Complete Yoga Breath."

The object of the exercise is to fill and empty the lungs very efficiently, thereby richly oxygenating the blood during filling and removing waste gases during emptying. The rhythmic quality of the breathing, over time, will bring about a heightened state of relaxation, inner peace, and healthy energy.

PROGRESSIVE RELAXATION

Have you ever noticed that you frown when you're worried or that your forehead wrinkles when you're faced with a difficult task? One of the things that happens to your body during times of stress is that your muscles become tense. This occurs because your body is preparing your muscles for action—to fight or to flee a perceived threat to your safety.

Progressive relaxation is a technique used to induce nerve and muscle relaxation. Developed by Edmund Jacobson, M.D., a physician who designed it for nervous hospital patients, the technique involves tensing one muscle group and then relaxing it, slowly moving from one muscle group to another until every muscle group in the body has been affected.

The purpose of first contracting the muscle is to teach people to recognize more readily what muscle tension feels like. The idea is to sense more readily when we are muscularly tense and then learn to relax. Studies show that learned relaxation of the big skeletal muscles that you have control over can affect the smooth internal muscles over which you normally have no conscious control. Learned relaxation can even help relax the cardiovascular system. Progressive relaxation has

The Complete Yoga Breath

1. Sit on the floor, with your legs crossed beneath you or in any comfortable position.
2. Make sure your back is straight (not arched or leaning forward), your head is erect and facing forward, and your arms are relaxed, with your hands resting on your thighs or on the floor.
3. Close your eyes and attempt to concentrate only on your breathing. Leave behind the worries or joys of your day and think only of this moment in time, when you are feeling the energy and power of your breathing.
4. Visualize your lungs as consisting of three parts—a lower space located in your stomach, the middle part near your diaphragm (just beneath your rib cage), the upper space in your chest.
5. As you breathe in through your nose, picture the lower space filling first. Allow your stomach to expand as air enters the space. Then visualize your middle space filling with energy, light, and air and feel your waistline expand. Feel your chest and your upper back open up as air enters the area. The inhalation should take about five seconds.
6. When your lungs feel comfortably full, stop the movement and the intake of air.
7. Exhale in a controlled, smooth, continuous movement, the air streaming steadily out of the nostrils. Feel your chest, your middle, and your stomach gently contract.
8. Make about four complete inhalations-exhalations in a minute, resting about two or three seconds between breaths. Rest for 20 seconds or so, then repeat the process until you feel more relaxed and in control.
9. As you perform this exercise, picture pure energy entering your body as you inhale, and visualize an outflow of impurities and tension as you exhale.

psychological benefits as well: Self-esteem is raised, depression lessened, and sleep problems alleviated in people who practice this relaxation method over a period of several weeks.

If you decide to use progressive relaxation, it is helpful to learn to recognize when you as an individual become most tense and where in your body the tension is centered. After you have more experience with progressive relaxation, you will be able to relax individual muscle groups from a standing or seated position. At the start, it may be best to work through your body, from head to foot.

Progressive Relaxation Exercise

1. Stretch out on the floor with your knees bent; make sure that the small of your back is on the floor so that you do not risk straining those muscles. If you like, support your head with a small pillow.
2. Take a deep breath and tighten the muscles of your feet by clenching your toes.
3. As you relax your feet, exhale. Notice the difference in the way your feet feel.
4. Breathe in again, and tighten the muscles of your calves. Hold the exertion for a few seconds.
5. As you exhale and release your calf muscles, say to yourself, "I feel relaxed."
6. Continue the process, with your knees, thighs, stomach, chest, arms, shoulders, neck, and face. Each time you tighten and release the muscles, feel yourself sink deeper and deeper into a state of relaxation.
7. When you have finished the process, breathe steadily and deeply for five minutes, enjoying the sense of relaxation.
8. Repeat the exercise daily for two weeks.

As you learn more about your body and the way it reacts to stress, you may be able to attain the relaxed state more quickly and directly. For example, you may be working at your desk and notice that your shoulder muscles are tense. To relax them you can tense them further, and then let them relax. When you focus on the warm, relaxed sensation of your shoulder muscles, you may feel your entire body, and spirit, relax as well.

BIOFEEDBACK

Biofeedback is one of the more scientific methods of revealing and measuring the mind-body connection. Its underlying premise is that high blood pressure—and other functions of the autonomic nervous system usually thought to be beyond conscious control—can be reduced if the person suffering from it learns to control the bodily responses involved. In other words, when properly trained, you can learn to lower your blood pressure and slow your heart rate by concentrating on doing so with your conscious mind. You will do so by triggering into action your parasympathetic nervous system to counteract the actions of your sympathetic nervous system during and after times of stress.

Biofeedback was developed when studies showed that animals could control their autonomic functions, like blood pressure, by being given a reward or a punishment. Physicians adapted those findings to design ways for humans to control, through conscious thought, what was once considered unconscious functions. Although there are several biofeedback methods, they all have three things in common: (1) they measure a physiological function (such as blood pressure); (2) they convert this measurement to an understandable form (a blinking light, mercury levels in a thermometer, etc.); and (3) thereby they feed back this information to the person learning to control his or her body processes.

One biofeedback method involves monitoring people with a machine equipped with lights similar to traffic lights. A special blood pressure cuff that has a microphone that will project the sound of any changes in blood pressure is attached to the patient's arm.

As blood pressure rises, the light on the machine, as well as the sounds being emitted by the microphone, lets the patient monitor the level of blood pressure. If it goes too high, for instance, the machine's lights may blink red. If pressure is normal, the light will turn yellow. If it's too low, it may blink green. The patient will learn to control his blood pressure by consciously calming down if the pressure is too high, or by thinking about stressful situations if the pressure is too low.

Although it sounds very mechanical, biofeedback is, in fact, a process that you can learn to master. The goal is to continue to control your blood pressure, pain from angina, or other symptoms of heart disease without the need for the monitoring machine. Over time, you would learn to recognize both the normally automatic physiological changes present with high blood pressure or, more likely, the stress that triggers it.

It is important to be guided through this process with the help of an experienced practitioner. If biofeedback interests you, talk to your mainstream or alternative practitioner about where and how to learn the appropriate techniques.

MEDITATION

Meditation is a mental exercise that affects body processes. It is used to filter out disruptive (stressful) thoughts and, by concentrating on a pleasant and calm image, word, or feeling, foster a sense of physical and mental relaxation. Meditation is effective both in reducing general stress and in directly improving the health of your cardiovascular system. As with other relaxation methods, meditation quiets the sympathetic nervous system, thereby reducing the heart rate, breathing rate, blood pressure, and muscle tension. These effects may last for hours after the meditation session.

In addition to its physical benefits, meditation can help you psychologically by allowing you to focus on the cause of your stress and to change the way you respond to the challenges you face. Researchers have found that by mastering meditative techniques, an individual can improve the sense of control over not only blood pressure but other aspects of one's physical and psychosocial life. Many people who meditate find that they are able to sleep more deeply, stop smoking more easily, and recover more efficiently from periods of stress.

Basic Meditation Exercise

This is a simple meditation exercise
that can help you relax and focus your attention
away from the things that cause stress
in your life. Start by sitting a few minutes—
perhaps just 5 to 10—until the practice
becomes comfortable to you.

1. Make sure you are wearing comfortable, loose, nonbinding clothing. Sweatpants or shorts and a T-shirt are ideal.
2. Find a quiet place where you will not be disturbed. Try not to sit any place where you might be easily distracted, such as in front of a window.
3. Sit on the floor in a comfortable position. If you can't sit on the floor, sit in a straight-backed chair.
4. Allow your hands to rest on your legs.
5. Lower your gaze so that your eyes are almost, but not quite, closed.
6. Take a deep breath and let it out slowly.
7. The easiest way to begin meditation is to count your breaths. Inhale, count one. Exhale, count two. Inhale, count three. Exhale, count four. Do this to ten, and then start again with one.
8. Sit for about 5 minutes every day for the first week or so (try timing yourself with a kitchen timer so that you don't have to keep track of the time). Gradually increase the time you meditate to 15, then to 30 minutes a day.

Although Christianity and Judaism also have similar traditions, meditation is largely grounded in Eastern cultures, particularly those of India and Tibet; you'll be learning more about it in Chapter 10, when you encounter Ayurvedic medicine. It is used as a method of spiritual awakening and as a form of religious ritual, as well as simply a way to relax the body and mind. There are many good books about meditation for you to choose from should you decide to use it as your primary method of relaxation (see *An Alternative Medicine Resource Guide*, p. 196). But the basic elements of meditation are very simple, and can be mastered by anyone willing to set aside a few minutes a day.

Meditation for relaxation requires no special training, and can be done at any time of day, and in any comfortable space. All it takes is several minutes to an hour of uninterrupted quiet.

Yogic breathing, progressive relaxation, biofeedback, and meditation are some of the best-known and most useful techniques for reducing stress. However, there are two others, one very common and one becoming more popular every day, that you may find helpful.

The first is one that, with any luck, you won't have trouble finding the time to do at least a little bit of every day: laughing. Although it has become a bit of a cliché, laughter truly is one of the best medicines known to humanity. On a purely physical level, it increases muscular activity, respiratory activity, oxygen exchange, heart rate, and the production of endorphins. These effects are soon followed by a relaxed state in which respiration, heart rate, blood pressure, and muscle tension rebound to below normal levels.

The psychological effects of humor are equally bountiful—it provides a healthy outlet for hostility, an escape from often unpleasant reality, and relief from anxiety and tension. If you can look at the world, and at yourself, with a bit of humor and a touch of whimsy, you'll find that your heart is not as heavy and your stress is not so great.

Another way to foster a sense of relaxation is through the use of scent, an emerging approach known as aromatherapy. Chapter 8 will show you how to use essential oils, made from flowers and herbs, to help you relax your body and mind.

"There is
no cure for birth
and death,
save to enjoy the
interval."

George Santayana

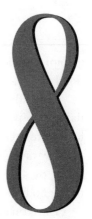

Aromatherapy

On your way to work one morning, you catch a whiff of lavender perfume wafting from the open windows of a neighborhood pharmacy. Almost immediately, you are awash in pleasant memories of your childhood. Transported back in time and space to your grandmother's home, where lavender sachets lined linen drawers and scented sheets covered the guest bed, you feel as warm and secure as you did when you were nine years old. By the time you arrive at the office, you feel more relaxed and calm than you have in weeks. If a doctor were to take your blood pressure, he or she might even find it lower than usual.

Although this example may not apply to you directly, no doubt you've experienced something similar. Perhaps the odor of a particular food evokes a feeling of comfort or the scent of certain flowers gives you energy. This strong connection between scent, emotion, and memory has led to a revival of an ancient form of medical intervention known as aromatherapy.

Aromatherapy is the branch of natural medicine that uses essential oils derived from the roots, stems, seeds, and flowers of plants to help restore emotional and physical balance to the body. First developed by the Egyptians some 5,000 years ago, aromatherapy is an offshoot of herbal medicine, which has been used in every culture throughout history.

The term aromatherapy was coined in 1937 by the French chemist René-Maurice Gattefossé, who badly burned his hand during a laboratory experiment in his family's perfume factory. Knowing that lavender was used in medicine for burns, he plunged his hand into a vat of pure lavender oil used to make perfume. After noting that his hand healed very quickly, Gattefossé began to explore the healing powers of other essential oils.

Essential oils, composed of the plant's most volatile constituents, are extracted from plants through a process of steam distillation or cold pressing. To derive pure essential oils, no other chemicals or substances should be used during the extraction process, since they would disrupt the natural organic composition of plant material. Indeed, each essential oil is made up of several different organic molecules that, working together, give the oil its unique perfume as well as its particular therapeutic qualities.

Like the plants and herbs from which they are extracted, some essential oils are known to have antiviral and antibacterial properties and thus can be used to treat infections such as herpes simplex, skin and bowel infections, and the flu. Other types of oils stimulate the anti-inflammatory response in the body, making them helpful in treating arthritis and similar conditions. Perhaps the most commonly used aromatherapy is one that uses oil derived from the eucalyptus plant which, when inhaled, works to restore health to the respiratory system by acting as an antibacterial, antiviral agent as well as an expectorant.

In this chapter, however, we'll be focusing primarily on the often profound effects that essential oils have on the central nervous system, and how those effects may impact on the cardiovascular system.

Aromatherapy and Heart Disease

As discussed in Chapter 7, one of the primary risk factors in the development of heart disease is excess stress. Stress overstimulates the sympathetic nervous system and the hormonal system, thereby raising blood pressure and heart rate and increasing blood lipid levels. Certain essential oils, when inhaled, can help to bring the sympathetic nervous system into balance with the actions of the parasympathetic nervous system and thus reduce the negative effects stress may have on the cardiovascular system.

How could an aroma have such a profound effect on internal body functions? To understand the answer to that question, it is important first to examine how the brain and the body recognize and react to scents. In effect, there is a pathway that brings scents from the air directly to your emotions. The pathway begins in the nose, where specialized nerve cells first recognize a scent, then pass the information on to other nerve cells. Finally, the sensory information is brought to a part of the central nervous system known as the limbic system.

One of the most primitive and least understood parts of the nervous system, the limbic system appears to be the seat of our emotions. It stores emotional information and memories that can be prompted by scent; once these emotions are triggered, they may set off physical reactions in the body, including a rise in blood pressure, heart rate, and serum cholesterol levels. By choosing essential oils known to help relax the nervous system, you may be able to help reduce the ill effects of stress on your cardiovascular system.

Using Aromatherapy

Essential oils are delicate, highly concentrated essences of plants. The quantity of plant material needed to make even a small amount of essential oil is enormous: To make an ounce of lavender oil, for instance, requires about 12 pounds of fresh lavender flowers. Fortunately, only a very small amount of oil is needed to have therapeutic effects.

Although it is possible to make your own essential oils with a homemade still, most people choose to purchase prepared oils from health-food stores and/or mail-order companies. (See *An Alterntive Medicine Resource Guide*, p. 196, for more information.) However, it is important that you make sure that the essential oils you use are just that: essential, meaning that their original chemical compositions were not altered in any way during the extraction process.

The fragrance industries, for instance, often use such toxic and irritating chemicals as hexane, methylene, and benzene to distill essences from flowers and plants. Although relatively harmless when used to make perfume, the essential oils extracted in this way have lost much of their healing qualities. When you purchase oils to use as aromatherapy, make sure they are labeled "Pure Essential Oils" or "PEO."

You can buy essential oils in their pure form or already diluted with another base oil, usually made from olives, soy, or almonds. In addition, herbs which "fix" the scents are added, so that the potency of the mixture is maintained over time. Combining essences with base oils does not change their chemical composition, but will help to reduce their potential toxicity to the skin or internal tissue. Although when used as directed the essential ingredients are safe, they can cause rashes, abdominal pain, and other unpleasant side effects. Always follow directions and/or consult an aromatherapist for information.

In general, there are two main ways to use essential oils as part of your stress management program to help prevent or reverse heart disease:

As inhalants. Simply breathing in the odors and minute particles of plant material will help bring your body back into balance. There are several equally effective methods of inhaling essential oils:

- *Aroma lamps*: Putting a few drops of oil on a light bulb or burning a candle under a cup that has drops of oil in it will volatilize the oil into the atmosphere, making your whole environment rich with soothing aroma.
- *Diffusers*: Mechanical devices disperse microparticles of essential oils into the air.
- *Facial saunas*: Pour boiling water into a bowl, then add a few

drops of essential oil. Drape a towel over your head and lean over the bowl so that the towel encloses both head and bowl. The essences are thus absorbed both through the skin and through the membranes of the nasal passages.

As topical applications. When diluted properly with base oils, essential oils may be safely and effectively applied directly to the skin.

- *Bath oils*: Adding a few drops of an essential oil to bath water both adds to the relaxing atmosphere and allows the oils to seep into the skin.
- *Massage*: Oils can be massaged into the face, back, chest, or any part of the body that is feeling pain or stress. Massage is an excellent relaxation method.

As is true of all forms of natural medicine, however, aromatherapy is highly individualized: An oil that relaxes one individual may work to stimulate another. Therefore, you may want to experiment by using a few different oils, alone or in combination, until you find one that works best for your needs. In addition, remember always that essential oils are, in fact, potent drugs and should thus be used with care. Discuss with your physician and/or natural medicine practitioner how aromatherapy can fit safely into your personal heart disease treatment plan.

Here are some other tips on aromatherapy:

- *Perform a patch test*. Before you use any essential oil on your skin, whether in the bath, as a liniment, or as a massage oil, make sure you first perform a patch test. To do so, wash about a 2-inch square area on your forearm and dry it carefully. Apply a tiny drop of the essential oil, diluting it with an equal part of a bland oil, like olive oil. Then place a Band-Aid over the area and wait 24 hours. If no irritation occurs, use the oil in the formulas. If you develop a rash or are otherwise made to feel uncomfortable, try another oil. A patch test is especially important if you have allergies or particularly sensitive skin.

- *Check with your doctor.* If you are pregnant, check with both your obstetrician and your alternative practitioner before using any essential oils. Do not take essential oils internally unless you first discuss the matter thoroughly with your practitioner.
- *Watch out for your eyes.* Keep essential oils out of your eyes.
- *Protect essential oils.* Store essential oils in dark glass or metal bottles and protect them from light and heat.

Aromatherapy for Heart Disease

Listed below are several essential oils considered beneficial to the heart and circulatory system. Again, however, you should check with your alternative practitioner before undertaking an extended aromatherapy regimen; essential oils are concentrations of powerful herbs and should be used with care. In addition, this list is far from comprehensive; if you are interested in exploring the world of aromatherapy further, check *An Alternative Medicine Resource Guide*, p. 196, for more information.

Angelica oil. Also known as the Root of the Holy Ghost, angelica oil is derived from a biennial plant whose roots and seeds are stem-distilled to produce a woody-scented oil. Most often used to help soothe indigestion and to heal scars and bruises, angelica oil is known to stimulate the circulation and remove toxins from the body.

Anise seed oil. Anise or aniseed is a tender annual that belongs to the same family as parsley and fennel; it is also known as sweet cumin. Originally grown in Asia, aniseed grows in both wild and cultivated states around the Mediterranean, and since colonial times has grown in the United States. Although the main property of anise is digestive, and it is used in Chinese and Indian medicine to treat indigestion, aniseed is also effective in calming heart palpitations.

Basil oil. Although first grown in India, the herb basil now is cultivated in many countries around the world, including the United States. Although we know it best as a cooking spice, basil is used in aromatherapy to fortify the nervous system and is an excellent remedy for anxiety or stress, especially when combined with soy oil and rubbed into the body.

Chamomile oil. Hippocrates, the ancient Greek physician often referred to as the Father of Medicine, dedicated the herb chamomile to the sun because "it cured agues." For centuries, chamomile and the oil derived from its flowers and roots have been used for medicinal purposes. Until World War II, chamomile oil was used as a natural disinfectant and antiseptic in hospitals and doctor's offices. It is known to help cure respiratory infections and allergies, as well as soothe indigestion, headaches, and menstrual cramps. Because of its relaxing effects, it is also helpful in reducing heart rate and blood pressure.

Clary sage/sage oil. Distilled from the flowering tops and leaves of a common perennial plant, chary sage oil has long been used for its medicinal properties. In fact, an aphorism from ancient Rome depicted sage this way: "How can a man die who has sage growing in his garden?" Chary sage oil is an all-around tonic that can help reduce fatigue, irritability, and depression and thus help to bolster self-esteem and reduce overall stress on the body.

Lavender oil. The classic oil of aromatherapy, lavender has a wide range of therapeutic qualities. Used topically, it can help heal burns, wounds, and insect bites. For patients with stress-related cardiovascular disease, it can work to bring the body back into harmony by calming the sympathetic nervous system and stimulating the parasympathetic nervous system.

Marjoram oil. Most often prescribed to reduce stress and anxiety, marjoram oil also increases circulation by dilating the arteries, making it a perfect choice for many people with high blood pressure.

Aromatherapy is one of the fastest-growing branches of alternative medicine in the United States. Please see *An Alternative Medicine Resource Guide*, p. 196, to locate organizations that can provide you with more information as well as discover the titles to some helpful books about aromatherapy. In the meantime, Chapter 9 explains the fundamentals of Chinese medicine and acupuncture as they relate to cardiovascular disease.

"Nature,

time, and

patience are

the three great

physicians."

Chinese proverb

Acupuncture and Chinese Medicine

9

*P*aul Jones, a 48-year-old man, came to me after having been diagnosed with borderline high blood pressure and early-stage coronary artery disease by a mainstream physician. A friend had suggested that traditional Chinese medicine might be a treatment option for him; Paul was particularly interested in finding out if acupuncture could alleviate his most obvious symptom, angina.

At the beginning of our first meeting, I made some observations about Paul's behavior and appearance. He had a rather tight, closed expression, and his face looked red and blotchy. He complained of having frequent hot flushes, especially in particularly warm rooms and during the summer. When asked how he felt about his health and his life in general, Paul admitted to feeling worried and a little depressed.

I then inquired about Paul's diet and exercise habits. He admitted to enjoying rich, fatty foods and indulging in alcohol more than he should; these habits had caused him to gain about 15 pounds over the past decade or so. He told me that he exercised fairly regularly and had stopped smoking several years before.

I had Paul undress and put on a gown, then began the physical examination. I started by carefully examining his tongue, noting that it appeared red, not pink, and puffy. I then took six pulses on each side of his body and felt along the meridians, finding areas of tension and sensitivity just below the breastbone and near the scapula. I palpated the abdominal organs noting that Paul's liver and kidney both felt tender. Finally, I felt Paul's neck and asked him to turn his head from side to side; I noticed that it was stiff. I observed, too, that Paul sometimes had difficulty forming words.

After Paul dressed, we sat together to discuss the diagnosis and the treatment options. I told him that his body was indeed in a state of imbalance that affected his blood pressure and his heart. In part, this imbalance was exacerbated by his eating and drinking habits, which were placing undue stress on his liver, creating an excess of liver yang. I also believed that he had a deficiency of qi affecting the heart, which contributed to his angina. I found, too, that his depression indicated a disturbance of the shen, the spirit that resides in the heart.

I suggested to Paul a treatment plan that involved acupuncture to relax the liver yang, build up the kidney yin, and free up the energy in the heart channel itself. I prescribed two herbal remedies, one called Xiao Yao San ("Free and Easy Wanderer") that works to cool out the hot, stuck energy of the liver and the other, Hu-po Yang-xin Dan ("Amber Nourishing the Heart Pill"), to strengthen the heart and stabilize the shen. In addition, Paul and I would perform a series of qigong exercises that work to build the qi and keep it moving freely through the body. I also recommended acupressure and other massage techniques. I told Paul that he would need to improve his diet, cut down on his drinking, and lose some weight.

Paul seemed relieved that he would probably not require surgery or drugs, but admitted that he knew little about Chinese medicine apart from what his friend had told him. Although I assured him *that the treatment would help bring his body into balance even if he did not completely understand the process, he would benefit even more if he took the time to explore the theory and practice of Chinese medicine. Six months later, Paul's blood pressure was in the normal range, his angina was infrequent, and, based on specialized x-rays, there were signs that his heart disease had begun to reverse. He also seemed more relaxed and open than he had when I first met him, and more ready to accept and contribute to the energy and joy in the world around and inside him.*

Medicine with a History

More than 2,500 years ago, a text known as *The Yellow Emperor's Canon of Internal Medicine* was compiled by an unknown group of healers in China. This first major treatise on Chinese medicine that has come down to us outlines an approach to life and health still practiced by more than one quarter of the world's population and followed, increasingly, here in the United States. It is a complex, all-encompassing philosophy based on Taoist tenets.

At its heart, the Chinese philosophy of health is based on the view that humanity, and each individual human, is part of a larger creation—the universe itself. Each of us is subject to the same laws that govern all of nature, including the stars, planets, animals, trees, oceans, and soil. In fact, Chinese medicine refers to the flows of bodily fluid and energy as channels and rivers and the state of the body as a whole in terms of the natural elements—dryness, heat, cold, dampness, wind.

According to Chinese philosophy, human beings represent the juncture between heaven and earth and thus a fusion of cosmic and earthly forces. Indeed, human beings *are* nature, and thus subject to its cyclic patterns and ebbs and flows, and the state of health of our universe, our planet, our individual bodies, is all connected through the same unified system known as the *Tao*. When any part of this unified whole becomes unbalanced, natural disasters (such as floods or droughts) or human disease may occur. What injures the earth injures each of us, and to heal the body is to foster the health and well-being of the whole universe.

Before you discover how heart disease is viewed in Chinese medicine and how you might benefit from seeking care from a practitioner of Chinese medicine, read the following overview of some general principles of Chinese philosophy:

YIN/YANG: INTERNAL BALANCE

In Chinese medicine, your health is determined by your ability to maintain a balanced and harmonious internal environment. Internal harmony is expressed through the principle of yin/yang, in which two opposing forces unite to create everything in the universe. Yin has connotations of cold, dark, and wet, while yang is bright, warm, and dry. Yin is quiet, static, inactive, while yang is dynamic, active, and expansive.

In a human being, Chinese medicine views parts of the body as having more yin or more yang qualities. The same is true of all physiological processes. Every organ of the body, for instance, is seen to be more yin or yang. The yin organs are the more solid ones—the heart, spleen, lungs, kidney, and liver. The more functional and hollow organs—the small intestine, stomach, large intestine, and bladder—are the yang organs. The organs work in mutual support and balance to maintain yin/yang balance within the organism as a whole. When yin/yang becomes unbalanced, then symptoms may occur, symptoms that we recognize as disease and ill health.

QI: THE LIFE FORCE

Another central principle of Chinese medicine is that health is maintained when energy, known as qi (pronounced "chee"), is allowed to flow unimpeded throughout the body. According to Chinese philosophy, qi is the energy essential for life. All the functions of your body and mind are manifestations of qi, and the health of your body is determined by a sufficient, balanced, and uninterrupted flow of qi. Qi ensures bodily function by keeping blood and other body fluids circulating to warm the body, fight disease, and protect the body against negative forces from the external environment.

Qi circulates through the body along a continuous circuit of pathways known as meridians. These meridians flow along the surface of the body and through the internal organs. When you are healthy, you have an abundance of qi flowing smoothly through the meridians and organs, which allows your body to function harmoniously and in balance.

HEART FACTS

Energy Medicine and Acupuncture

Current research performed in the United States links the effectiveness of acupuncture to the electrical currents that run through the human body—currents that are measured by such well-known diagnostic procedures as the ECG (electrocardiogram) and the EEG (electroencephalogram). Scientists have discovered that the traditional Chinese system of meridians and acupuncture points are remarkably accurate in locating the energy flow through the body, giving a modern slant to the ancient concept of Qi.

If qi becomes blocked along one of your meridians, on the other hand, the organ meant to be nourished by this energy will not receive enough qi to perform its functions. By locating where in the body qi is blocked, and by releasing it, Chinese therapists attempt to restore proper energy flow to the body. For example, angina, a major symptom of heart disease, is often felt in the arm, along the heart meridian.

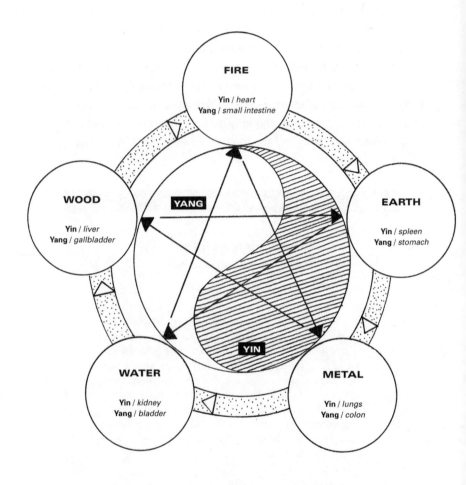

*According to the Chinese tradition of medicine and health,
all apsects of ourselves and the universe are held in an intricate state of
balance that if upset may result in disease or disharmony.
The yin and yang and Five Phases, depicted above, show the relationship
between the seasons of the year, the parts of our bodies,
our emotions, and even qualities of temperature, color, and taste.*

THE FIVE PHASES

Another component of Chinese medicine is called the Five Phases theory. This theory provides a coherent structure to the flow of qi and the balance of yin with yang. This system places all natural phenomena into five categories, each of which represents a stage in the annual progress through the seasons. The five categories are wood (spring), fire (summer), earth (late summer), metal (autumn), and water (winter). Linking the seasons of the year, aspects of nature, and the body's organs, the Five Phases reflect the ever-changing and diverse aspects of nature while providing a unified structure to the universe.

As the illustration shows, the meaning of the Five Phases is best understood as a creative cycle, with each phase nourishing and promoting the activities of the next. In your body, each of the five seasons relates to one yin and one yang organ: Spring is associated with the liver (yin) and gallbladder (yang), summer with the heart (yin) and small intestine (yang), late summer with the spleen (yin) and stomach (yang), autumn with the lungs (yin) and large intestine (yang), and the winter with the kidneys (yin) and bladder (yang).

Visiting a Chinese Doctor or Acupuncturist

Like most other natural medicine modalities, Chinese medicine provides no standard diagnostic signs or treatment plans. Instead, each patient is evaluated based on his or her own unique constitution and energy level. Essentially, Chinese doctors attempt to treat disease by restoring yin/yang and a healthy qi flow to the body. In general, three forms of treatment are used, often in combination: herbs, acupuncture, and an exercise program known as qi-gong. Later in this chapter, these three treatments will be explained in more detail. In the meantime, let's explore what you might experience if you decide to visit a practitioner of Chinese medicine.

Many Americans used to Western medical techniques and technologies are surprised by the kind of examination they receive from someone who practices Chinese medicine. Far more time than usual is spent discussing the symptoms that prompted you to visit a doctor in the first place—perhaps a desire to lower your blood pressure or alleviate the pain of angina—as well as aspects of your life and lifestyle that may be relevant to your general health.

For instance, the doctor may well ask you how you feel about or react to heat and cold, dampness and dryness, seasonal variations, and day-to-night changes in mood and feelings of well-being. Other questions may concern bowel movements, menstruation, and eating and drinking habits. Your answers to the questions will give the doctor an idea of what part of your system is out of balance and what kind of treatment you may need to return to a state of internal harmony.

A PHYSICAL WITH A DIFFERENCE

The physical examination is quite different from what you might expect, too. A Chinese doctor places a great deal of importance on listening to your pulse. In fact, he or she will feel twelve different pulses, six on each side, and each related to a different organ in your body. The pulses also relate to meridians—energy pathways through the body.

Your Chinese doctor may also spend time looking at your tongue, which, according to the tenets of Chinese medicine, reveals much about your body by its coating, its color, and its shape. By examining your tongue, the doctor is also attempting to locate where in your body qi flow has been disrupted. The abdomen also is important in some acupuncture systems, and therefore a Chinese practitioner may press on points in the stomach to feel for tenderness, warm or cool areas, and a pulse in the umbilicus (belly button). Finally, your Chinese doctor will feel along the meridians for signs of tenderness, temperature changes, and other irregularities in the tissues.

Chinese Medicine and Heart Disease

In Chinese medicine, most cases of heart disease can be traced to a problem in the liver meridian. In fact, the liver is called "the mother of the heart." (Chinese doctors hold that problems in one organ often originate in its mother organ.) However, other cases may be caused by a depletion of kidney energy. Since the kidney signifies water and the heart fire, a depletion of water will lead to a problem with too much fire, affecting the heart. A third type of cardiovascular problem involves the heart energy itself. Since the heart holds the spirit in Chinese medicine, depression or other emotional upset can stir up this spirit.

Because the nature of Chinese medicine is extraordinarily individual, it is impossible to say what your particular diagnostic procedure might be like. Returning to the case history at the beginning of this chapter, though, we can see how a diagnosis of heart disease and high blood pressure can be made using the principles of Chinese medicine.

Our patient, Paul Jones, seemed angry and tightly controlled, indicating that his liver qi was constrained or blocked. His red, swollen tongue and his tight, wiry pulse confirmed this. The heart, kidney, and fire pulses were weak, he had some pressure of speech, and he was tender in the heart and kidney areas, around his sternum and his upper back, signifying the weakness of heart qi and the chronic nature of the problem, which has exhausted the kidney qi. Finally, his depressed outlook and expression suggested that the shen, the spirit, was unhealthy.

In Paul's case, I chose to treat his problems with a combination of all three forms of Chinese therapy: acupuncture and massage, herbal medicine, and qi-gong, or energy-releasing exercise.

ACUPUNCTURE AND MASSAGE

Throughout the body, there are over one thousand "acupoints," areas that can be stimulated to enhance the flow of qi. When special needles are inserted into these points, they help correct the flow of energy and thus restore health. The actual point of insertion depends on the site of the disorder and the way in which the therapist wishes to influence the qi. The insertion of the very thin needle should be nearly painless, although there is a mild pinprick as the skin is pierced. Care is always taken to avoid blood vessels and major organs.

Acupuncture needles may be inserted to a depth of about one-fourth to two inches or more, depending on a variety of factors, including the patient's size and the part of the body concerned. The needles are left in place for a few seconds up to an hour; the average time is about 20 minutes. Along with needles, moxibustion is often used to warm and tone the body's qi. Special herbs called moxa and derived from the herb mugwort are heated either above or on a specific acupoint.

In Paul's case, I chose to move the "stuck" liver qi by inserting needles in liver and gallbladder points on the feet, dispersing the stuck energy and moving it into the heart. In subsequent treatments I would strengthen the heart by using points on the fire meridians of the arm, and their connections to the chest and the back. Moxa on these points warms the heart and corrects its deficiency of qi. Special points around the sternum and inside the wrist correct the disturbance of shen. Finally, strengthening the kidney with points on the abdomen and legs helps build reserves of energy.

HERBS

The use of herbs is an essential part of traditional Chinese medicine. They are used to reorganize the body constituents (qi, blood, and body fluids) within the meridians and the internal organs, as well as to help the body adjust to the impact of any external forces.

In general, Chinese herbal medicine involves using multiple herbs in combinations that have specific effects. One combination used to treat heart disease (and which I prescribed in Paul's case) is called Xiao Yao San ("Free and Easy Wanderer") and works to cool the stuck energy of the liver. In addition to these combinations, herbs can be added according to specific symptoms. For instance, diuretic herbs, like the fungus *Poria cocos*, may be prescribed to someone whose high blood pressure is related to water retention.

Herbs are dispensed in many different forms, including pills, tinctures, powders, and capsules. Fresh herbs may also be given, and people must boil them in water then drink the strained liquid. Herbs are usually taken over a period of one to two weeks.

QI-GONG

A third form of Chinese therapy is qi-gong, which literally translates to mean "energy exercises." Qi-gong builds the qi and helps to move it freely around the body. These exercises work to cultivate inner strength, calm the mind, and help maintain the body's natural state of internal balance and harmony or, if upset, restore the balance.

There are several different types of qi-gong. Some exercises are similar to calisthenic or isometric movements, others are meditative stances, still others involve the stimulation of acupressure points through massage. Breathing exercises, similar to those described in Chapter 7, are designed to bring the body into a state of relaxation and harmony.

The basic qi-gong posture involves standing with your feet apart, your knees slightly bent, your back straight, and your arms held in front of your body. You are then to imagine that you are holding an imaginary "ball of qi" in front of you. This posture is maintained from a few minutes to a half-hour, and will improve your circulation, warm your hands, and relax you.

For heart problems, in particular, there is a heart qi-gong, which consists of using your right palm to massage over the left part of your chest, in a circle covering the left breast, while silently repeating the sound "Ho." This form of massage may also be done by a qualified acupuncturist, who will be using his or her own qi to move and release your qi.

Finally, there are massage points to help angina and heart attacks (between the 7th and 8th vertebrae in the spine), for heart failure (the kidney points along each side of the sternum), for high blood pressure (at the outside of the elbow crease), and for arrhythmias (three finger widths up from the wrist crease on the inside of the arm). Although

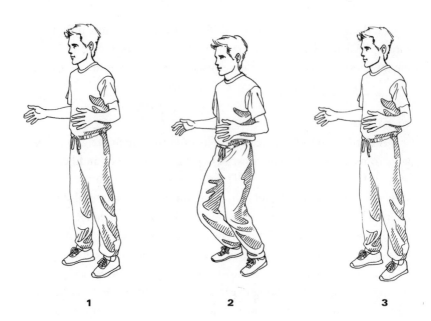

1   **2**   **3**

*Qi-gong is an acient Chinese exercise that stimulates
and balances the flow of qi, or vital life energy, along the energy
pathways in the body. One basic qi-gong posture,
pictured above, is designed to help you hold and control energy
within and outside of your body. 1) Stand straight, with your
palms facing, and take a full breath. 2) Bend knees and squat
down a bit. As you exhale, say the syllable, "choo."
3) Slowly stand, return to starting stance, completing your inhalation.
Repeat the exercise.*

massage and acupressure can easily be learned for self-care, it is important that you first learn the technique from a qualified acupuncturist.

Acupuncture licensing requirements are different in each state. Some states license only M.D.'s to do acupuncture; other states require separate licenses for acupuncturists. Licensed acupuncturists should have taken a national certification or equivalent exam and physicians should have completed a minimum of 225 hours of training—the amount set by the World Health Organization.

The end of the twentieth century appears to be an exciting time for medicine here in the United States and around the world. As the precepts of traditional Chinese medicine, with its emphasis on self-care and internal harmony as a way to ensure health, become better known and understood, we'll have less need for the often expensive high-tech surgical and pharmaceutical options. And we'll be able to enjoy the best of both worlds, East and West.

In Chapter 10, you'll learn about another system of thought, one developed in India, that also looks at health and disease within a holistic and natural framework.

"Man is the epitome
of the universe.
There is in man as much
diversity as in
the world outside, and
there is in the
world as much diversity
as in man."

Ayurvedic tenet

Ayurvedic Medicine

10

$\mathcal{T}$wenty-five hundred years ago, in the fifth century B.C., a philosophy of health known as Ayurveda developed in India. Today, millions of people around the world base their understanding of well-being on these ancient teachings. Indeed, the Sanskrit word Ayurveda means "the science of life and longevity."

Like its cousin, traditional Chinese medicine, Ayurvedic medicine sees each individual person as an extension of the universe, and health as a state of balance within the body and between the body and the universe. In Ayurveda, as in most holistic forms of health and healing, there is no dividing line between body, mind, and spirit, and disease can be caused by physical, psychological, or spiritual imbalances. If one's mind and spirit are in harmony, the body will be healthy as well. But if the consciousness is filled with conflict, the physical self will descend into disease. In this view, all disease involves both physical and spiritual factors and thus requires treatment on both levels.

Ayurveda also holds that all of life—including disease—consists of learning and the development of self-knowledge. In this way, disease is seen as an opportunity to reexamine our spiritual and physical lives in order to correct imbalances and bring us back into alignment with the energy of nature and the universe. Disease, therefore, is a healthy way to bring us closer to what is known as the cosmic consciousness.

The Principles of Ayurvedic Medicine

The life force, which is known as qi in Chinese medicine, is called "prana" in Ayurveda. Prana is the animating power of life, providing vitality and endurance to each human being. Ayurveda also teaches that within each of us is a divine healer, a cosmic consciousness, that if properly directed can restore balance and energy to the body. Treatment of disease in Ayurvedic medicine seeks to strengthen and direct an individual's cosmic consciousness.

Balance and harmony are maintained by what is known in Ayurvedic medicine as the *three doshas*—forces of energy that act on the substances and organs within the body. When the three doshas are balanced, the body can function harmoniously, resulting in good health. When the three doshas become imbalanced, disease is created.

THE THREE DOSHAS AND METABOLIC TYPE

Although we all have elements of each of the three doshas within ourselves, Ayurvedic tradition believes that each individual also has a specific body type, also called a dosha. Your dosha is determined by your body shape, personality, and many other qualities of body function. Once your dosha is determined, your Ayurvedic practitioner can prescribe the right kind of diet, exercise, and daily routines to keep you in optimal health. Since a prime goal of Ayurvedic medicine is preventing disease from occurring in the first place, understanding one's own dosha and practicing a lifestyle designed to maintain dosha balance becomes important.

Although each person's metabolic type is determined by a predominant dosha, all three doshas are present in everyone and in every cell of the body. In general, a balance among the doshas will create a state of vitality in which the physical, emotional, and intellectual qualities are balanced. It is important to remember that the doshas are factors of both physical and psychological disease. An unbalanced dosha or doshas create emotional or mental disorders as well as physical problems.

In fact, the main cause of disease in Ayurveda is said to be "failure of intelligence," or *prajnaparadha*. Prajnaparadha is a lack of understanding of the natural harmony of life and how to adapt to it, which often results from fear, desire, greed, or other destructive forces that keep us from trusting in the divine consciousness to bring peace and balance to our existence.

Below are short descriptions of each type of dosha as it applies to body type:

Vata (pronounced vah-tah) represents the force of kinetic energy within your body. It activates the physical system and is responsible for breathing and the circulation of blood. The seats of vata are the large intestine, pelvic cavity, skin, ears, and thighs. Organs associated with vata include the bones, the brain (especially motor activity), the heart, and the lungs (in the act of breathing).

If you are predominantly a vata body type, you tend to be rather thin, with prominent features and cool, dry skin. You may have a rapid speech pattern and a feeble pulse. Vatas tend to be moody and vivacious and have active, creative minds. They keep irregular hours, and are especially prone to anxiety and disorders of the vata organs. Vata's season is autumn—a dry, windy season during which vata people tend to develop arthritis, rheumatism, and constipation.

The *kapha* dosha is responsible for physical strength and stability. It holds together the structure of body and is located in the chest, lungs, and spinal fluid. Organs associated with kapha include the brain (primarily information storage), joints, lymph, and stomach. If you have a predominantly kapha body type, you tend to be heavyset

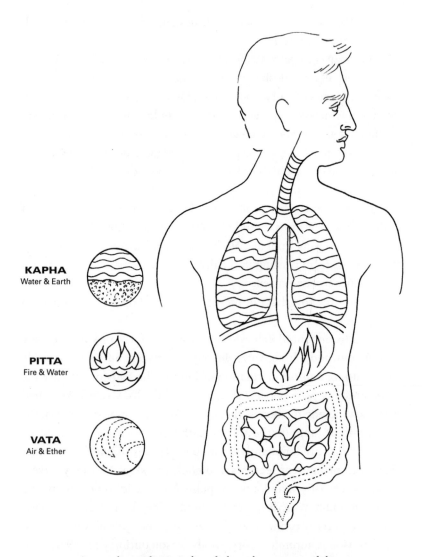

KAPHA
Water & Earth

PITTA
Fire & Water

VATA
Air & Ether

Ayurvedic medicine is founded on the concept of three distinct metabolic body types called doshas. *Aspects of these different body types, known as* vata, pitta, *and* kapha, *are believed to exist within every individual in specific areas of the body, as depicted in the diagram above.*

and have cool, oily skin. Kaphas are often very relaxed and tolerant people, who are slow to anger but have a tendency to procrastinate. They sleep for long hours and may eat not for the physical but rather for the emotional pleasure that food brings to them. Kapha types are especially prone to obesity, and thus to heart disease, as well as to illnesses of the kapha organs, such as allergies and sinus problems. The kapha season is winter, when the respiratory system is particularly susceptible to colds and congestion.

Pitta governs the metabolic processes of cells. Organs associated with pitta include the blood, the brain (especially memory and learning), hormones (when stimulating activity), liver, small intestine, and spleen. If you're a pitta body type, you tend to have a medium build, thin hair, and warm, ruddy skin. Pittas are organized, work hard, and have very regular sleeping and eating habits; their need for structure may tend toward perfectionism. Although generally warm and loving, a person with a predominantly pitta dosha may also display quick bursts of temper. Pittas tend to suffer from acne, hemorrhoids, and ulcers, and may often feel warm and thirsty. The pitta season is summer, when the heat and bright light may aggravate pitta-related disorders, including rashes, diarrhea, and other inflammatory conditions.

PRINCIPLES OF DIAGNOSIS AND TREATMENT

As is true in many forms of alternative medicine, the process of diagnosis in Ayurvedic medicine relies far more heavily on the practitioner's powers of observation and questioning than on laboratory tests and imaging techniques. If you're like most Americans who are more familiar with Western techniques, you may be surprised when the Ayurvedic practitioner begins to smell and touch your skin in order to examine all aspects of your body and personal behavior. Don't be alarmed, however; this is how your condition will be diagnosed and a treatment plan devised.

Your examination will probably begin when the Ayurvedic practitioner takes your pulse. In fact, he or she will listen to your pulse at twelve separate sites on the wrists—six on the right wrist,

six on the left. Measuring the pulses informs the practitioner of the
movement of prana—energy—through the body and the general
health of each internal organ.

Another important diagnostic tool used in Ayurvedic medicine, as
well as in traditional Chinese medicine, is the examination of the
tongue. According to Ayurvedic tradition, each area of the tongue is
related to a different organ in the body; and by observing the surface
of the tongue, the practitioner can tell many things about the internal
order or disorder of the doshas. A whitish tongue, for example, indicates an imbalance of kapha and a black discoloration indicates a vata
disturbance in the organs represented by the areas on the tongue.
You'll probably be asked to provide urine and feces samples as well.

In addition, your Ayurvedic practitioner will ask you a great
many questions about your past medical history, your present symptoms, and your general feelings about your personal life and physical
condition. Not only will your practitioner take note of *what* you say,
but also the *way* you speak: the strength and the sincerity of your
voice (or the lack of it) may reflect your willingness to accept responsibility for your own health.

Based on the results of these and other examination procedures,
an Ayurvedic doctor will identify dosha imbalances and the diseases
that result from them. After diagnosis, a treatment plan is developed
that has as its primary goal the removal of the original cause of the
disease and thus the reestablishment of dosha balance.

All treatment involves the use of food and nutrition, herbs, yoga
exercises, meditation, massage and essential oils, and breathing exercises. You may be asked to begin treatment by *detoxifying* your body
of impurities or toxins that are often the result of undigested, unab-
sorbed food. Detoxification may consist of induced vomiting, ene-
mas, blood cleansing (by bloodletting and using blood-thinning
herbs), and nasal douching. Next you might be asked to perform certain yoga, chanting, and meditation exercises, a process known as
palliation. Palliation also often involves lying in the sun for long
periods of time. Taking certain herbs that stimulate healing is also
included in this stage.

After the cleansing regimen, the Ayurvedic practitioner may prescribe for you a period of *tonification*. During tonification, you'll consume certain herbs and perform particular yoga, meditation, and breathing exercises. Another step in the Ayurvedic method of healing involves mental and spiritual meditation, called *satvajaya*. Satvajaya has as its goal the reduction of psychological and emotional stress, as well as the release of negative emotions and ideas.

Ayurvedic Medicine and Heart Disease

In Ayurvedic as well as Chinese medicine, the heart, not the brain, is the seat of consciousness. For that reason, heart disease often reflects any deep-seated issues of identity, feeling, and consciousness that we hold inside of us. Causes of heart disease, according to Ayurvedic tradition, may include a wrong diet, physical or emotional trauma, suppressed emotions, and/or excess anxiety.

Heart disease can occur with any of the three doshas. Vata heart disease is indicated by palpitations and tightness in the chest and a feeling of restlessness, fear, and anxiety. People who experience pitta heart disease may feel flushed, may have nosebleeds, and may vomit sour fluids. Psychologically, people who have pitta heart disease feel angry and irritable and may suffer bursts of temper that aggravate other symptoms. Kapha types, on the other hand, may experience heart disease as a heaviness in the chest, may develop a stubborn cough, and are often tired. These people are also likely to feel stubborn, acquisitive, and unable to let go of emotions.

Treatment of all types of heart disease in Ayurvedic medicine is completely dependent upon the emotional, spiritual, and physical attributes of each individual. Some general prescriptions include:

Relaxation and meditation. Since the heart is the seat of consciousness and spiritual energy, the first step toward health should involve a period of physical, spiritual, and emotional rest. You may find, as many people do, that meditation and yoga exercises will help bring you back in touch with your true heart's desires.

Detoxification. The first step in this process is to eliminate cigarette smoking, alcohol, and as many environmental pollutants as possible. Other detoxification methods, like those described above, should be undertaken with care and only under supervision.

Diet. In addition to prescribing a diet that will help restore your particular dosha imbalance, an Ayurvedic practitioner is likely to recommend that you eat foods rich in antioxidants, such as vitamins C and E and beta-carotene. They are especially likely to recommend adding onions and garlic to your diet. Furthermore, your general diet will be assessed and recommendations made based on your specific dosha.

Herbal remedies. There are a number of herbs that may help strengthen your heart; again, a practitioner will recommend different herbs depending upon your specific dosha imbalance and its suspected cause.

Like its cousin, traditional Chinese medicine, Ayurvedic medicine is a comprehensive and complex philosophy involving far more than simple diagnosis and treatment for any particular disease. To choose Ayurvedic medicine as a way to treat your heart disease would most likely involve looking at your body and your spirituality in a whole new way, and require that you make significant changes in your eating and exercise habits as well as in your spiritual outlook. If you are unfamiliar with Ayurvedic philosophy, you need to explore the subject far more thoroughly before making such a decision. (See *An Alternative Medicine Resource Guide*, p. 196, for resources.)

In Chapter 11, we'll explore another type of holistic alternative. In chiropractic, the focus is on the proper alignment of the spine and joints as the means to health and vitality.

"Practice not -

doing and

everything will

fall into place."

Lao-Tzu

11

Chiropractic
Medicine

$\mathcal{B}$est known as a treatment option for lower back pain and other musculoskeletal disorders, chiropractic now ranks as the second largest primary health care field in the world, with more than 15 million people in the United States visiting a chiropractor every year. In addition to its usefulness as therapy for muscle- and joint-related disorders, chiropractic therapy has proven to be an effective complementary treatment for a wide range of other ailments, including high blood pressure and heart disease.

Chiropractic therapy centers on restoring proper balance and structure to the spinal column and joints. And, by doing so, it restores proper working order to the nervous system, which radiates from the spinal cord to the organs and tissues of the body. When the spinal cord is misaligned, it prevents the nervous system from transmitting messages to the muscles, organs, and tissues which, in turn, are unable to function as they should. Pain and/or disease may result.

Chiropractic theory holds that by keeping the spine in alignment through regular visits to the chiropractor and through proper exercise, you will help your body carry out all of its functions, including healing itself of most ailments. Chiropractic, then, can be seen as both treatment for injury and illness and a method of preventing disease.

Chiropractic Diagnosis and Treatment

The spinal column is made up of twenty-four bones, called vertebrae, that surround the spinal cord, a sheaf of nerve tissue reaching from the base of the skull to the upper part of the lower back. Coming from between the vertebrae are pairs of spinal nerves that extend out to every part of the body. Included among these nerves are those of the sympathetic and parasympathetic nervous systems, which help control functions such as heart rate and blood pressure.

According to chiropractic theory, when vertebrae become misaligned—through trauma, stress, and chemical imbalances, among other things—pressure is placed on the nerves in the affected area. Messages to and from those nerves are distorted and the body's ability to function smoothly and in harmony is disrupted. Any change in the normal function of the vertebrae, and of the nearby nerves, can have a wide range of effects on the entire body. Chiropractors attempt to correct the misalignments, which they call *subluxations*, to allow the body to function properly once again.

When you visit a chiropractor, he or she will first attempt to make a diagnosis of your condition by taking a detailed case history and giving you a physical examination. In fact, a chiropractor's diagnostic procedure begins as soon as you come through the office door and he or she notices the way you walk, stand, and sit. Your eating and exercise habits will be assessed and the chiropractor will ask you questions about your symptoms. During the next part of the exam, you'll probably be asked to bend forward, backward, and sideways, and to rotate your spine. These exercises help the chiropractor to measure the range of movement of your spine and extremities. Your reflexes will also be tested so the chiropractor can asses nerve function. The chiropractor will probably feel your spine and various other joints—a process known as palpation—to further assess mobility. Under certain circumstances, x-rays may be required to derive more information or to confirm a diagnosis.

Once you are diagnosed, your chiropractor will help you develop a treatment plan. Treatment focuses on adjusting the subluxation by mobilizing and manipulating your spine. Mobilization may be both active, in which you stretch your body in a certain way, or passive, in which the chiropractor assists the movement, stretching your spine (or whatever joint is being treated) past its range of passive movement to achieve an adjustment. Another process, known as the high-velocity thrust, involves the chiropractor placing his or her hand on a particular vertebral area and then thrusting forward with a certain amount of force and speed. The technique used to achieve an adjustment is determined by the chiropractor based on your own particular needs and physical constitution.

Chiropractic and Heart Disease

Generally speaking, the causes of heart disease include genetic, environmental, and lifestyle factors that go far beyond the capacity of chiropractic therapy to alleviate. A chiropractor would most likely refer a patient with high blood pressure, coronary artery disease, and/or angina to a physician for evaluation and treatment. He or she may also recommend a nutritionist, herbalist, or other alternative therapist for additional support.

However, chiropractic has proved to be a useful complementary treatment for cardiovascular disease in several different ways: First, proper alignment of the spine allows the autonomic nervous system to function properly. The two branches of the autonomic nervous system, the sympathetic and parasympathetic, must work in coordination with each other and with the hormonal system in order for normal blood pressure and heart function to be maintained. The part of the spine most involved with cardiovascular function is the upper cervical region, located in the neck.

Second, adjustment of the midthoracic region of the spine (located in the middle of the back) frees the nerves that stimulate kidney function, helping the body eliminate salt and water through more efficient urine production. This lowers blood volume and, hence, blood pressure. Manipulation of the midthoracic region also has an effect on the biochemical activities of the adrenal gland, leading to increased production of the hormone aldosterone. Aldosterone is essential to proper salt and water retention and excretion.

Finally, by releasing areas of tension held in the spine, chiropractic promotes general relaxation. As stress reduction is an essential part of any successful cardiovascular treatment plan, chiropractic is especially useful to anyone with cardiovascular disease.

Again, although chiropractic is not recommended as a first-line treatment strategy for most people who suffer from coronary artery disease and/or high blood pressure, it is certainly worth exploring as part of an overall holistic plan to bring your body back into its natural state of balance.

Chapter 12 addresses another type of holistic medicine, one that focuses on the healing power of herbs.

"Man argues,

nature acts."

Voltaire

Herbal
Medicine

12

$\mathcal{T}$he most ancient form of health care known to mankind, herbal medicine has been used in all cultures and throughout history. Even today, approximately 25 percent of all prescription drugs in the United States are derived from trees, shrubs, or herbs; many other drugs are synthesized to mimic a natural plant compound.

In general, herbal medicines work in much the same way as conventional pharmaceutical drugs. They contain a large number of naturally occurring chemicals that work within the body to alter the body's own chemistry. Unlike purified drugs, however, plants contain a wide variety of substances and, hence, less of any one particular active chemical. This attribute makes plants far less toxic to the body than most pharmaceutical products.

Another benefit of natural herbs is that they tend to contain combinations of substances that work together to restore balance to the body with a minimum of side effects. An example is the plant meadowsweet, which contains compounds similar to the ones used in aspirin that act as antiinflammatories. These compounds, called salicylates, often irritate the stomach lining. Unlike commercially prepared aspirin, however, meadowsweet also contains substances that soothe the gastric lining and reduce stomach acidity, thus providing relief from pain while protecting the stomach from irritation.

Most important, like other forms of alternative therapy, herbal medicine attempts not to cure disease per se, but rather to help the body remain in, or return itself to, the state of balance we know of as health. In attempting to restore health, the herbalists explore lifestyle and dietary habits with their patients to develop an individualized treatment plan. They carry this exploration far beyond where most mainstream physicians would go.

Herbal remedies form an important part of many other types of traditional approaches to medicine and health, including Chinese medicine and Ayurveda. Although these systems share a common goal—the restoration of internal harmony—each may use herbs in a slightly different way, depending upon how the body is viewed and the condition diagnosed.

That said, there are some generalities we can make about the way different herbs act on the body and how they may be used to treat specific illnesses. Some herbs act best as antiinflammatories, soothing the symptoms of inflammation or reducing the inflammatory response of the tissue directly. Others are known to be effective antimicrobials, helping the body destroy or resist bacteria and viruses. Still other herbs are best used as stimulants for the digestive system.

Herbs may be used as part of a holistic approach to the treatment of heart disease that includes proper nutrition, exercise, and stress reduction. Herbs that might help the body restore the cardiovascular system to proper working order include those known to be hypotensive (blood-pressure-reducing), diuretic (fluid-reducing), calmative (anxiety-reducing), and tonic (energy-building).

It cannot be stressed enough that there are no set prescriptions in herbal medicine or in any form of alternative therapy. As is true for any dietary program, nutritional supplement plan, or exercise routine, herbal treatment of your particular heart condition must be designed with care by a trained professional who has taken the time to examine you. In addition, it is up to you to learn as much as possible about your body, your health, and the herbs prescribed by your practitioner.

HEART FACTS

Of the 250,000–500,000 different kinds of plants growing on the earth today, only about 5,000 have been studied for their medical applications.

In fact, one factor herbalists take into consideration when diagnosing and treating a patient is that person's willingness to accept responsibility for his or her own health.

At a first appointment with an herbalist, you should expect the practitioner to take a complete medical history (including noting what medications and supplements you are taking) and possibly perform a physical exam. The herbalist would then prescribe one or more natural medications aimed at strengthening your constitution while alleviating your symptoms.

Herbs are available in many forms including the following:

- *Whole herbs:* Plants or plant parts that are dried and either cut or powdered to be used as teas or as cooking herbs.
- *Capsules and tablets:* A fast-growing corner of the herbal medicine market are capsules and tablets, which allow herbs to be taken quickly and without requiring you to taste them.
- *Extracts and tinctures:* Extracts and tinctures are made by

grinding the roots, leaves, and/or flowers of an herb and immersing them in a solution of alcohol and water for a period of time. The alcohol works both to extract the maximum amount of active ingredients from the herb and to act as a preservative.

The Herbal Medicine Chest for Treatment of Heart Disease

Herbal medicine can become an effective part of an overall cardiovascular treatment plan. A qualified herbalist should be able to help you devise a healthy diet, suggest nutritional supplements, and discuss with you the need to increase your physical activity and reduce the number of stressors in your life. Likewise, most herbalists work well with other health care professionals, from both mainstream medicine and other alternative therapies. It is important, however, that *all* of the people who care for you are apprised of any treatment you receive.

Make no mistake about it: Herbs *are* drugs, and powerful ones at that. Let your herbalist know what medications you are taking and if you are pregnant or breastfeeding so that he or she can create a safe and effective herbal treatment plan for you.

Although your particular body chemistry will indicate what herbs will be most effective for you, the following herbs are the ones most used to treat cardiovascular disease:

FIRST-TIER CHOICES

Hawthorn (*Crataegus oxyacantha*). The berries, flowers, and leaves of the hawthorn shrub have been used in folk medicine in Europe and China for centuries and are some of the primary heart tonics in natural medicine. More recently, medical researchers have analyzed hawthorn extensively and studied it for its different effects on the cardiovascular system. Hawthorn berries (as well as most other berries) get their color from substances called flavonoids. Flavonoids, besides being potent antioxidants, dilate coronary blood vessels, lower blood lipids, and stabilize arterial walls. They also act to inhibit an enzyme, ACE, which helps create high blood pressure. In fact, they function similarly to the drug captopril, commonly given to combat high blood pressure. Because hawthorn improves heart muscle metabolism, it is useful in treating congestive heart failure and cardiac arrhythmias. It's also mildly diuretic. This versatile herb can be used, alone or in combination with other herbs, to both prevent and treat the whole spectrum of cardiac illnesses.

Preparation and usage: Dried hawthorn berries or flowers, 3 to 5 grams, can be taken as capsules or teas three times per day. Standardized fluid extracts (infusions) can be taken, ¼ to ⅓ teaspoon three times per day. Hawthorn has a low toxicity.

Garlic (*Allium sativum*). The volatile, sulfur-containing oils that give garlic its pungency also are known to reduce LDL cholesterol (the bad kind) and raise HDL cholesterol (the good kind). In Germany, garlic extracts are approved over-the-counter drugs to supplement dietary measures in people with elevated blood lipids. And in India a study matching two populations with identical diets except for garlic showed lower blood lipids in the high-garlic group. Garlic and its close relative onion have also been shown to aid in thinning the blood and reducing platelet aggregation, helping to minimize the risk of blood clots that could clog an artery in the heart or brain. Finally, garlic has lowered blood pressure by 10 to 20 points in both human and animal studies.

Preparation and usage: In studies that showed the benefits of garlic, researchers used 3 to 8 cloves of raw garlic daily. Capsules are also available; unfortunately the substance responsible for many of garlic's good effects, called allicin, is also responsible for its strong odor, and capsules with the substance removed do not work as well as whole, fresh garlic. There is some evidence that capsules coated so that they break down low in the intestines work better, and with less odor. About 2 to 6 capsules per day is a common dose.

Ginkgo biloba (*Ginkgoaceae*). The leaves of this tree, the oldest species in the world, contain special flavonoids which give the plant both its characteristic smell and some of its remarkable vascular effects. Ginkgo has been shown to increase arterial blood flow successfully in a variety of situations, including cerebral vascular insufficiency and stroke, in hardening of the peripheral arteries, in impotence due to lack of blood flow, and in cardiac problems. Ginkgo also keeps blood platelets from sticking and breaking down, and it increases oxygen supply to the arteries and veins.

Preparation and usage: Standard preparations of *ginkgo biloba* extract (GBE) are usually 40 milligrams and are taken three times a day. Higher dosages are not recommended.

Guggul (*Commiphora mukul*). The Indian mukul myrrh tree produces a resin which has been shown in multiple studies to lower cholesterol and triglycerides as well as or better than the common drugs on the market, and with no known toxicity. It works by increasing the liver's metabolism of LDL cholesterol.

Preparation and usage: The common form of gugulipid is an extract with 4 percent guggulsterone (the active component); standard dosage is 500 milligrams taken three times per day. (The standard preparation contains 25 milligrams of the active ingredient per dose.)

Coleus (*Coleus forskohlii*). This decorative plant has been used in India for centuries and studied in detail for its cardiovascular effects. It relaxes smooth muscles, which makes it useful in treating high blood pressure and angina. At the same time, it increases the force of heart contractions so that the net result is a double positive effect.

Preparation and usage: The dose is the same as for hawthorn, and the two herbs are frequently used together to treat cardiovascular conditions. Coleus has very low toxicity.

SECOND-TIER CHOICES

Ginseng (*Panax ginseng*). The herb ginseng, over which wars have been fought in the Orient in past centuries, is actually several different substances. Korean or Chinese ginseng (*Panax ginseng*) is the famous one, and is known to reduce blood clot formation, reverse oxidation, and lower blood lipids. It also has a paradoxical effect on blood pressure, seeming to raise blood pressure in low doses and lower blood pressure in higher doses. But the main use of ginseng is in helping to cope with stress, primarily by improving adrenal gland function.

Siberian ginseng (*Eleutherococcus senticosus*) shares the effects of improving adrenal function and lowering lipids. In addition, it seems to bring both high and low blood pressure closer to normal ranges.

Preparation and usage: One of the most popular ways to consume either type of ginseng is by drinking it as a tea or infusion made by stirring about ½ teaspoon of powdered ginseng into a cup of hot water. The tea should be drunk about three times a day. Standard fluid extracts (1:1) can be taken, ½ to 1 teaspoon, three times a day. A visit to a Chinese herbal pharmacy will reveal Chinese ginseng roots to be as expensive as $200 or more per piece, and this price is related to the potency (amount of active substances). A reasonably priced root ($10 to $15 range) can be sliced into 2 to 6 gram pieces (about 2 square inches) and cooked as tea. Too much high-quality ginseng can be toxic.

Ginger (*Zingiber officinale*). Ginger lowers cholesterol, and has a tonic effect on the heart.

Preparation and usage: Ginger can be cooked in foods, made as a tea, or taken as capsules 2 to 3 times a day.

European mistletoe (*Viscum alba*). This herb is a potent treatment for high blood pressure. In Europe there are many blood-pressure-lowering herbal preparations containing mistletoe on the market.

Preparation and usage: This herb can be toxic and is usually used in small amounts (½ to 1 teaspoon of the dried herb) combined with hawthorn and other herbs.

Bilberry (*Vaccinium myrtillus*). This berry is rich in the same flavonoids as hawthorn and has many of the same effects. Bilberry seems to be particularly helpful in strengthening the circulation; it has been used extensively in treating varicose veins and thrombophlebitis.

Preparation and usage: Bilberry is nontoxic and may be used liberally, dried in tea or fluid extracts in the doses given for hawthorn.

Khella (*Ammi visnaga*). This plant has been shown to be effective in the treatment of angina and high blood pressure. An article in the

New England Journal of Medicine in 1951 supported its use in angina pectoralis. Khella appears to be particularly helpful in increasing the amount of exercise a person can tolerate before experiencing angina.

Preparation and usage: Standard doses would be 250 to 300 milligrams of the extract (containing 12 percent of the active component khellin). Higher doses may cause side effects. The herb may be used with other herbs for heart treatment.

Angelica (*Angelica archangelica*). The various species of angelica can be used to treat angina, high blood pressure, lack of circulation to the brain and the limbs, and arrhythmias. Angelica can easily be grown in a home garden, as long as the soil is kept moist and the area is shaded during the hottest part of the day.

Preparation and usage: Angelica is usually prescribed in the same dose as khella and has low toxicity.

Cayenne (*Capsicum annuum*). Usually thought of only as a hot spice in Mexican and Southwestern cuisine, cayenne is also one of the most effective general tonics for the body. It stimulates blood flow and strengthens the heartbeat.

Preparation and dosage: To make an infusion of cayenne, pour a cup of boiling water onto ½ to 1 teaspoon of the herb and let it stand for 10 minutes. A tablespoon of this infusion should be mixed with hot water and drunk.

Chamomile (*Anthemis noblis*). Perhaps the best known and most widely used herbal medicine, chamomile is used most commonly to promote relaxation and reduce stress in people with heart disease. (See Chapter 8 for information about chamomile and aromatherapy.)

Preparation and dosage: Chamomile tea is made by pouring a cup of boiling water over two or three teaspoonsful of dried leaves and letting it stand for five to ten minutes.

Foxglove (*Digitalis*). The plant from which the widely used cardiac medication called digitalis comes, foxglove is now considered too dangerous to be used at home. Unless your medical herbalist is trained to use this substance, foxglove should be avoided.

In Chapter 13, you'll read about another approach to the treatment of disease that uses herbs and other natural substances in a very different way, an approach known as homeopathy.

"The highest ideal of cure is the speedy, gentle, and enduring restoration of health by the most trustworthy and least harmful way."

Samuel Hahnemann

Homeopathy

13

*H*eart disease and high blood pressure are usually considered chronic conditions that develop largely as a result of long-term deficiencies or excesses in our lifestyle—poor diets, lack of exercise, high stress levels—that cause our bodies to become unbalanced. As such, they are perfect examples of "modern diseases" that can be successfully treated by holistic therapies that involve working to restore proper balance to an individual's own internal environment.

Homeopathy, a branch of holistic medicine, is an example of such a therapy. If you think you might be interested in exploring homeopathy as part of your treatment, it is essential that you first learn all you can about its philosophy and methods before you make a decision. Above all, you should not stop taking any cardiovascular medication until you first check with your mainstream physician and/or consult with a qualified homeopath.

The ABCs of Homeopathy

Late in the eighteenth century, German physician Samuel Hahnemann developed a new system of medicine, one that broke away from the emerging modern pharmacy and operating rooms that were fast becoming the mainstays of Western medicine. The system he developed came to be known as homeopathy, derived from the Greek work *homoios* (meaning "similar") and *pathos* (meaning "suffering"). Today, the World Health Organization estimates that some 500 million people around the world now use homeopathy as a treatment for disease.

Hahnemann, a deeply spiritual man, believed that a physician's role should be to help a patient's own body heal itself and that true healing could not take place by simply administering chemicals that would, in essence, override the body's natural processes. Inside every human, Hahnemann believed, was a "vital force," a life power that animates and rules the body, keeping it in balance and health. Disease occurs when a disturbance of this vital force takes place.

What we think of as symptoms of disease homeopathy views as the external evidence of the vital force's internal attempts to bring the body back to a state of balance. To a homeopath, a "disease" consists of the symptoms produced by the body in its own efforts to heal itself. To help the body in that process—to strengthen the vital force against the illness—a homeopath administers remedies designed to match these symptoms, not to alleviate them as Western medicine is designed to do.

This principle is known as Hahnemann's *Law of Similars*, or "like cures like." By making symptoms temporarily worse, a remedy would be strengthening the body's own power to heal itself. In fact, in the view of homeopathy, any therapy that attempts to suppress the free flow of symptoms will actually prolong the underlying disturbance, since it prevents the body from being able to heal itself.

Another theory of homeopathic medicine is known as the *Law of Infinitesimals*. First developed by Hahnemann in order to reduce the side effects of often potentially toxic chemicals, this theory states that the smaller the dose of medicine, the greater its potency and its effect on the body's vital force. Homeopathic remedies are extracts derived by soaking plant, animal, mineral, or other biological material in alcohol to form what is known as the *mother tincture*. This tincture is again diluted with alcohol in ratios of one part tincture to 10 or 100 parts of alcohol, shaken vigorously, then diluted again.

This process of shaking and diluting, repeated several times, is known as *succussion*. Many researchers believe that through succussion the vital energy of a substance is transferred to the tincture. Therefore, the more times the solution passes through succussion, the more potent the remedy, even though there appears to be no trace of the original herb or mineral left. Finally, the resulting solution is added to tablets, usually made of sugar, and then is ingested by the patient.

Prescriptions for homeopathic remedies are written only after a homeopath carefully evaluates a patient's particular set of symptoms and physical and emotional makeup. Indeed, a session with a homeopath may be a unique experience for those of us who are accustomed to Western medicine's approach to diagnosis and treatment. A homeopath will spend much more time talking to a patient about symptoms and lifestyle factors, and look more carefully at demeanor, personality, and coloring, than will a mainstream physician.

In fact, the way that a homeopath treats a disease depends entirely on an individual's particular pattern of symptoms. Not everyone with angina, for instance, experiences chest pain in exactly the same place, at the same time, or for the same reasons. While a conventional, mainstream physician will offer the same treatment to almost everyone (usually beta blockers or calcium-channel blockers), a homeopath recognizes several different symptom patterns associated with angina and has corresponding remedies for each one. The symptoms of the individual are matched with the pattern of symptoms produced by a remedy; the more closely the remedy matches the total pattern of the patient, the more effective the remedy will be.

Furthermore, the symptoms that first bring a patient to the doctor (called *common symptoms* in homeopathy) are rarely the most important symptoms when it comes to selecting a remedy. Instead, *general symptoms*, which include the patient's state of mind and mood, are given more weight in determining a treatment. Other symptoms, called *particular symptoms*, are those that pertain to any given organ (angina, for instance). They, too, are less important than the general symptoms. Most important of all are what homeopaths call *strange, rare, and peculiar symptoms*; as their name implies, they are symptoms that are completely unique to the individual describing them. A man who says that his blood feels like it's boiling and a woman who feels as if she is made of glass and easily broken are examples of two people with strange, rare, and peculiar symptoms; even if each of them also experiences chest pain, they would probably be given different remedies.

In addition, an important aspect of homeopathy is the *Law of Cure*, which postulates that symptoms disappear in the reverse order of appearance. In other words, the last symptoms to appear will be the first to disappear with treatment. If a patient has had many health problems in his or her life, he or she may find that symptoms of past problems reappear as homeopathic treatment continues. Someone who comes to a homeopath for angina, for instance, may find that he or she briefly develops symptoms of bronchitis, a previous illness. Slowly but surely, working backward in time, the homeopathic remedy or remedies will restore strength to the vital force and balance to the internal environment.

Homeopathy and Cardiovascular Disease

It is impossible to describe how a homeopath would diagnose or treat a person with cardiovascular disease, since therapy is based completely on individual needs and symptoms. In fact, a homeopath may not consider the source of cardiovascular disease to be the heart or the vessels themselves at all, but rather an imbalance elsewhere in the body or mind. Like many other forms of holistic medicine, homeopathy sees the emotional and intellectual health of an individual as being as important—in fact, as being more important—a factor in physical health.

According to homeopathic tenets, mental and emotional disturbances are more serious than physical illnesses, primarily because they can themselves cause physical disease. Heart disease is a perfect example: Mainstream Western medicine acknowledges that high stress levels and the emotions they provoke (such as anger, anxiety, and irritability) are directly linked to high blood pressure and coronary artery disease.

Because treatment is dependent on symptoms, any of the several hundred homeopathic remedies described in Hahnemann's *Materia Medica Pura*, upon which modern homeopathy is based, might be prescribed. Very generally speaking, however, homeopathic remedies for cardiovascular disease might include the following:

- *Aconitum napellus*: Also known as wolfsbane or monkshood, this perennial herb contains aconitine, which is a deadly poison. When succussed to a homeopathic dose, however, aconitum appears to slow the pulse and calm the breathing, making it a suitable treatment for individuals whose cardiovascular disease may be due to excess stress.
- *Arnica montana*: So named because it grows in the mountains of Europe and the northwestern United States, this herb is known to reduce high blood pressure and to help resolve other heart disorders.
- *Belladonna*: Also called deadly nightshade, belladonna contains atropine, a potent central nervous system stimu-lant. Belladonna may be prescribed to a patient with high blood pressure.
- *Calcarea carbonica*: Calcarea is made from oyster shells and has a high calcium content; as such, the remedy is often indicated when the calcium metabolism is imbalanced, thus affecting the blood pressure.

The homeopathic treatment of any disorder, including cardiovascular disease, requires ongoing observation and, in some cases, a series of different remedies prescribed on the basis of new, emerging symptoms. Fortunately, the remedies tend to be relatively inexpensive and, once a person's condition and makeup are well understood by both the homeopath and the individual himself or herself, may be self-administered at home.

It is important for you to thoroughly research the subject of homeopathy and how it might be useful in treating your cardiovascular disease *before* you decide to no longer seek treatment from a mainstream physician. Chapter 14 will discuss some of the guidelines you should follow in making such a decision, as well as answer questions you may have about any of the holistic, alternative methods explored in this book and how they apply to the understanding and treatment of cardiovascular disease.

"Have the courage to live. Anyone can die."

Robert Cody

Developing an
Alternative Plan

....

*Y*ou've now had a chance to read about the many alternatives to surgery and drug therapy available to treat heart disease and high blood pressure. Although the options may seem confusing and occasionally contradictory, they all have the same goal in common: to bring your body into a natural state of balance so that your heart and blood vessels can function properly.

Although one type of alternative therapy may place greater or lesser importance on certain foods, herbal and other remedies, and types of exercise, any successful treatment of cardiovascular disease will involve the following:

- Maintaining a healthy weight
- Cutting down on fat in the diet

- Reducing negative physical and emotional stress
- Bringing your body back into balance through exercise and meditation

Nevertheless, there are significant differences in philosophy between various alternatives. Deciding which alternative is best for you is a highly personal decision, one that may involve investigating several different options before committing to one or another treatment plan.

In the meantime, take a look at the following ideas about how to use and choose an alternative health care method:

Use holistic medicine as a preventive tool. The best time to explore a new form of treatment is not during a health crisis, but rather when your body is in a state of relative good health. If you know that cardiovascular disease runs in your family, it is never too early to make sure that your body is in balance by following a holistic approach to health. In that way, you may be able to prevent an acute crisis, like a stroke or heart attack, before it occurs.

Invest in some bibliotherapy. A fancy name for learning through reading, bibliotherapy is essential in order for you to gain a thorough understanding of the various philosophies of health and disease—before you decide how you would like to address your particular cardiovascular problem and your general health.

Work with a mainstream physician who is willing to explore options with you. As we move toward the twenty-first century, more and more of medicine is bound to include the best of both mainstream and alternative options. If your physician is willing to learn, but does not know much about these options, you can share your resources, inlcuding this book, with him or her. If you are currently being treated by a physician who is not open to other philosophies and methods, you may want to consider choosing another doctor more sympathetic with your needs.

Live well and in harmony with the universe. If after you've read this book, you decide not to pursue an alternative form of medical care, you still should attempt to open your heart and mind to the natural flow of energy, within and outside of your body. Reread Chapter 7 to learn how to meditate and thus become more in tune with your inner desires, or Chapter 6 on exercising outdoors so that you can observe, and take part in, the rhythms of nature.

The rest of this chapter is devoted to answering some of the questions my cardiovascular patients have asked me and my colleagues, not only about heart disease but also about the various treatment options described in this book. We hope that the answers provided address some of your own questions and concerns.

Understanding Heart Disease

Q. I'm 56 years old, with a family history of heart attack, and my blood pressure is at 180/100. My doctor wants to put me on medication, but I'm afraid that if I start taking drugs, I'll have to take them for the rest of my life. I have about 20 pounds to lose, and I just stopped smoking. Could I solve my problem without drugs?

A. In the long run, you might be able to control your high blood pressure without medication. However, right now you're blood pressure is in the danger zone for someone with your family history of heart attack. With the addition of your weight problem and history of smoking, your doctor is probably right to put you on medication immediately. However, it is quite possible that once your blood pressure is controlled and you've lost the weight, your doctor may slowly wean you from the medication. However, *do not* stop taking your medication without first consulting your physician.

Q. So far, my blood pressure is normal, but high blood pressure and cardiovascular disease run in my family. Should I worry about my children's blood pressure?

A. It's never too early to instill healthy habits that will help your children avoid high blood pressure. If you have a family history of high blood pressure or heart disease and have children, it is important to monitor their blood pressure and fat intake carefully. By instilling proper diet and exercise habits in your children from a very young age, you could help prevent them—as well as yourself—from developing cardiovascular disease later in life.

Q. I've been diagnosed with high blood pressure and I also am overweight. Which is more important to control if I want to avoid having a heart attack?

A. Quite frankly, that's a difficult question to answer since both may have an equal impact on your heart. Luckily, however, you may be able to kill two birds with one stone: If you lose weight by cutting saturated fats and sugars out of your diet, your blood pressure is likely to drop at the same time. Obesity is one of the most important risk factors for high blood pressure, and therefore for heart disease. Many of the same foods that lead to obesity also will tend to raise the blood pressure and lead to heart problems. If you lose weight and your blood pressure drops, you're that much farther along the road to cardiovascular health.

Exploring the Options

Q. Why are synthetic drugs, like the beta blockers I take for high blood pressure and angina, considered bad for me by most alternative health practitioners?

A. Man-made drugs, also called pharmaceuticals, are not necessarily considered "bad for you"; in fact, some drugs may be veritable lifesavers under certain circumstances. Nevertheless, pharmaceuticals usually focus on alleviating symptoms, not on addressing underlying problems. They also tend to take over body functions rather than help the body to work properly on its own. Finally, drugs often produce unpleasant side effects—side effects that, in essence, only add to the state of imbalance that caused the original symptoms to occur. Choosing herbal remedies that attempt to restore the body to proper working order while producing a minimum of side effects is often a much safer alternative.

Q. I've had two heart attacks and two bypass operations. I'm very interested in finding a healthy alternative to drugs and surgery and have been reading about the many different options, particularly traditional Chinese medicine. But I've never been a religious person and the emphasis on a spiritual force that helps us heal bothers me.

A. Spirituality is a belief that we are connected to and dependent upon something outside ourselves, whether that something is nature, each other, or the unknown. It is important to distinguish this from religion, which is a specific belief system that defines and explains that connection. Although Eastern healing systems stem from philosophical and religious beliefs, it is perfectly possible to derive benefits from these systems without subscribing directly to the philosophy. What is important is a belief that you have the power to control your health and your future, and that you can do this by altering the external world (by diet, stopping smoking, exercising, and changing stressful situations) and the internal world (by not holding onto emotions, by learning to relax, to love and to play, and by encouraging hope and positive thoughts). Perhaps, through this process, you'll also find a new way to address spirituality in your life.

Q. Is it possible to cure or at least control heart disease by diet or exercise alone?

A. Because the causes of heart disease—indeed, of any chronic disease—are varied and complex, it is unlikely that changing just one aspect of your life will lead you to cardiovascular health. By far, learning to eat well and exercise often are the most important methods of alleviating heart disease. However, bringing your body into a true state of harmony involves not only addressing nutritional deficiencies or excesses, but also examining your emotional and spiritual state and working to find inner peace. That's why a holistic approach, as embodied in traditional Chinese or Indian medicine, is a good choice for many people with cardiovascular disease.

Choosing an Alternative

Q. I have been diagnosed with early-stage coronary artery disease, and I want to see a homeopath. My mainstream physician objects strongly. What should I do?

A. That's a delicate question without an easy answer. Many mainstream physicians, who are reputable and highly qualified, find it difficult to accept the tenets of homeopathy. You should discuss the matter thoroughly with your doctor to find out if he or she would still treat you even if you decided to visit a homeopath on a regular basis. Perhaps the homeopath would be willing to speak to your physician or provide material regarding the extreme safety of homeopathy. If your doctor refuses, then I would suggest that you find a new mainstream physician, one who is more willing to explore other treatment options with you.

Q. I've had two heart attacks and know that I'm alive today thanks to the high-tech medical care I received at the hospital after those events. I want to explore alternatives, but I don't want to give up on what has worked for me in the past.

A. There is no doubt that modern medical technology saves lives, especially during acute crises like heart attacks and strokes. Nevertheless, modern medicine has its own set of limits, including its lack of attention to prevention and its frequent inability to address the root causes of illness.

Fortunately, we are living in a time when high-tech medicine and its holistic counterparts are learning to work in cooperation with one another. We live in a country in which many options are available to us at the same place and time. You'll still have access to the lifesaving diagnostic and medical therapies you feel work for you while investigating holistic options.

Diet and Nutrition

Q. I've changed from eating butter to eating margarine. Is margarine any less fattening or better for me?

A. No. Butter and margarine each contain equal amounts of calories. However, margarine has artificially constructed fats, called transfatty acids, which are harmful to the arteries and make it a poor choice for people anxious to prevent heart disease. The healthiest diet uses very little fat; I don't object to my heart patients using a pat of butter here or there, although I encourage people to experiment with the Italian custom of using olive oil—a much healthier choice than either butter or margarine—on their bread and pasta.

Q. I'm supposed to be cutting down on sodium because of my high blood pressure. Is garlic salt and/or sea salt okay to use?

A. That depends. Research has shown that only a small percentage of people are actually salt-sensitive. If you and your doctor have determined that sodium causes your body to become imbalanced, then the use of flavored salts would not be recommended because they contain the same amount of sodium as regular table salt. Sea salt, which contains less sodium and more of the important minerals magnesium and potassium, may be a better choice. However, traditional Chinese and Ayurvedic medicine may look differently at the way your body functions, and you may discover that salt is not a problem for you when your body is truly in balance. In the meantime, you may want to try using flavored *peppers*, such as lemon pepper, or other spices.

Q. I love to eat fish and hear that it's a good source of protein and pretty low in fat. Am I right?

A. As long as you don't cook your fish in fat or load it with heavy cream sauces or dressings (like tartar sauce), you've made an excellent choice for your heart and for any weight loss efforts you've embarked upon. Not only does fish tend to have less fat than meat, but the fat that is in fish is highly polyunsaturated, which means that it does not raise blood cholesterol levels. Moreover, fish fat contains a special group of polyunsaturated fatty acids known as omega-3s, which have been shown to protect against heart disease by reducing the ability of the blood to clot. Blood clots that travel to coronary arteries are a leading cause of heart attacks. Omega-3's also lower levels of triglycerides, another type of fat implicated in cardiovascular disease. Fish especially high in omega-3's include salmon, mackerel, herring, sardines, tuna, and anchovies.

Exercise and Your Heart

Q. I know that exercise is an important part of any treatment for heart disease, but I also know that exercise can cause heart attacks in susceptible people. I have high blood pressure, and heart attacks run in my family. Do I exercise or not?

A. Before you start any exercise program, get your doctor's permission. If your condition is serious, he or she may recommend very mild and short periods of exercise for a number of weeks—say, walking at a slow pace for ten minutes—until you build up some cardiovascular endurance. Your doctor will probably recommend that you have a stress test performed at various intervals to test the strength of your heart. However, starting and sticking with an exercise plan will definitely increase your cardiovascular health, and your general sense of well-being, over the long term.

Q. I'm always reading that to get any benefit from exercise, you should work at your target heart rate for at least 20 minutes. Is that necessary?

A. Not at all. Recent research has shown that performing any exercise, for any length of time, is beneficial to your heart and your body in general. Simply taking the stairs instead of riding the elevator, and walking to the market instead of driving, will help you keep your cardiovascular system healthy. On the other hand, working at the level you describe is the most efficient way to build cardiovascular endurance and to burn fat. If you want to get into tip-top shape, you may decide to work toward reaching and maintaining your target heart rate for about 20 minutes at least three times per week.

Q. I always thought that yoga was a meditative technique, but my gym is offering what they call "aerobic yoga." Is there such a thing?

A. Yoga is used as both a form of exercise and a method of attaining a higher state of consciousness through proper breathing and meditation. The beauty of yoga exercise lies in its ability to bring the body into balance through quiet, powerful stretching and by focusing the student on his or her breathing to bring more oxygen into the body. Unfortunately, your gym instructor may lose sight of these benefits in an attempt to get the heart rate up by forcing you to move through the postures more quickly than usual. Although it's difficult to advise you without knowing more about the class, I would tend to think you should find another type of aerobic activity and enjoy yoga for its ability to strengthen and stretch your body.

Stress Reduction and Aromatherapy

Q. I've been diagnosed with high blood pressure and when I get angry I can feel my heart start to beat faster, my palms start to sweat, and I feel agitated. Is my blood pressure higher at this point than at others?

A. Perhaps, but remember, high blood pressure means that your blood vessels and heart are working harder *all the time*, not just when you're angry or upset. In fact, it is natural for blood pressure to rise at times of stress and then to return to a normal healthy level when the crisis is over. If you've been diagnosed with high blood pressure, it means that your blood pressure is elevated all the time. However, your anger and frustration level may indicate that you feel under constant pressure and stress and have found no healthy ways to release the tension that results. Read Chapter 7 for more information.

Q. Every night after I get home from work, I spend five to ten minutes writing down everything that I have to do the next day and all the things that are bothering me. I think it helps me relax, but my wife claims that it only makes my problems seem more important than they are. Who's right?

A. More than likely, you are. A study at Pennsylvania State University showed that people were able to reduce their anxiety levels by setting aside a "worry period" every day. If they started to fret about their problems or future tasks at other times in the day, they forced themselves to postpone it until that period. The organization such a system provided gave the subjects a feeling of control that calmed them down. I'd say you were on the right track.

Q. Is aromatherapy only used for relaxation or do the herbs from which oils are derived have physical effects as well?

A. First of all, it's important to realize that relaxation *is* physical. More and more evidence is surfacing every day that emotion, and thus the effects of emotion, are present in every cell of the body, including the heart and blood vessels. Second, there is some evidence that therapeutic particles of the original plants enter the body through the nasal passages and the skin and work internally the same way as a dose of herbal medicine by mouth would work.

Chinese Medicine

Q. I have been to an acupuncturist who used a lot of needles, and left them in a long time. My friend went to another acupuncturist who used very few needles, and just stuck them in and out. What is the difference?

A. There are several different systems of acupuncture being practiced in the United States, depending on the acupuncturist's training. Chinese-style (Traditional Chinese Medicine), as you experienced, tends to use several needles which are retained. Japanese style uses a more gentle stimulation and fewer needles, and French style, favored by many physician-acupuncturists, is somewhere in between. It is best to discuss the system with the acupuncturist prior to or at the first appointment.

Q. I would try acupuncture, but I'm worried about AIDS. Is this a risk with acupuncture needles?

A. In this era of AIDS awareness, it is highly likely that your acupuncturist is using disposable, single-use acupuncture needles. In addition, all acupuncturists licensed by the National Commission for the Certification of Acupuncturists (NCCA) are required to take clean needle training as part of their examination for licensure. Even so, it is important to ask your prospective acupuncturist if he or she uses disposable needles.

Ayurvedic Medicine

Q. Ayurvedic medicine involves the idea that we have a cosmic consciousness that we can control and that can control our health; that sounds a little like the "power of positive thinking." Is it the same thing?

A. In a way. The most important common element in all forms of alternative therapy is the belief that the body has the power to heal itself and that you are able to direct that power on a conscious or spiritual level. Ayurvedic medicine calls this power the "cosmic consciousness," but it is known by different names in other cultures and traditions.

Q. Ayurvedic medicine seems very elaborate and multilayered. How much do I have to understand before I can start to heal my heart disease?

A. Learning about your body from an Ayurvedic perspective is a process, one that may take many years, indeed a lifetime, to go through. An Ayurvedic practitioner will guide you through that process while providing you with practical information about proper diet, exercise, herbal medicine, and meditation techniques. If you follow this advice, you should see positive change in the state of your health relatively quickly, probably within a period of several weeks, depending on your condition.

Chiropractic and Your Heart

Q. I've been seeing a chiropractor for a lower back injury, and my doctor has told me that my blood pressure, which had been on the high side, is now normal. Could there be a connection?

A. Absolutely. Depending on where on the spine your chiropractor is working to alleviate your lower back problems, therapy may be helping to reduce your blood pressure in one of two ways. If your chiropractor is concentrating on your neck area, it's likely that he or she is helping to balance the activity of the sympathetic and parasympathetic nervous systems in the function of the heart and blood vessels. The midback area, on the other hand, is connected to kidney function; it is likely that your kidneys are producing more urine, or the adrenal glands, which sit atop the kidneys, are producing a hormone that helps to lower blood pressure.

Q. What kind of training does a chiropractor usually have?

A. To be certified as a chiropractor, an individual studies at a chiropractic college for a minimum of four years. Training includes all of the basic science and diagnostic skills taught to a medical student, but does not involve surgical or pharmaceutical study. Some chiropractors learn the fundamentals of nutrition as well.

Herbal Medicine

Q. I'm taking high blood pressure drugs prescribed by a mainstream physician, but I'm interested in beginning to treat my cardiovascular disease with herbs. Can herbs interfere with the drugs I'm taking?

A. Herbs *are* drugs, and yes, if your physician and herbalist do not work together—or are not at least aware of how each is treating you—you could run into some problems with the effectiveness of your treatment plan. It's up to you to supply all the people who treat you with a list of any and all medications and remedies you are taking.

Q. I'm allergic to penicillin and a variety of antibiotics. Could I be allergic to herbal remedies as well?

A. Absolutely, and you must be sure to inform your herbalist of any and all allergies and sensitivities you may have to drugs and other substances. This information will help him or her provide you with a safe, effective herbal remedy.

Homeopathy

Q. I'm not sure I understand the way homeopathy works, and what I do know makes me unsure that it really does work, but I have friends who swear by it. Do I have to believe in it for the therapy to work?

A. Having faith that a treatment has the potential to work is certainly helpful, but it is not necessary for you to fully understand homeopathy to reap its benefits. In fact, many homeopaths are unsure themselves exactly how a substance diluted so many times still has the power to heal. Nevertheless, millions of people around the world find relief from a variety of ailments with homeopathy, and you may be able to do so as well.

In the next chapter, we offer some of the vast resources available to you in your quest for a safer, more effective, and longer-lasting approach to healing your heart.

An Alternative Medicine Resource Guide

··

$\mathcal{T}$he world of alternative medicine is opening up to Americans more and more every day. Following is a list of associations and organizations that provide information on all aspects of their particular field—from lists of qualified practitioners to explanations of the finer points of their philosophies and approaches to health and disease. Books, pamphlets, and videotapes are often available, sometimes at no cost, sometimes with a fee. In addition, we have provided a brief bibliography listing some of the hundreds of new and older books that you can read to find out more about all aspects of alternative medicine.

Acupuncture/Chinese Medicine

American Academy of Medical Acupuncture
5820 Wilshire Boulevard, Suite 500
Los Angeles, CA 90036
(800) 521-AAMA

American Foundation of Traditional Chinese Medicine
505 Beach Street
San Francisco, CA 94133
(415) 776-0502

National Commision for the Certification of Acupuncturists
1424 16th Street, NW
Washington, DC 20036
(202) 232-1404

National Oriental Medicine and Acupuncture Alliance
636 Prospect Avenue
Hartford, CT 06105
(203) 232-4825

Qigong Institute/East-West Academy of Healing Arts
450 Sutter Street
San Francisco, CA 94108
(415) 788-2227

READING LIST

Beinfeld, Harriet, and Korngold, Efrem. *Between Heaven and Earth: A Guide to Chinese Medicine.* New York: Ballantine Books, 1991.

Kaptchuk, Ted. *The Web That Has No Weaver: Understanding Chinese Medicine.* New York: Congdon and Weed, 1992.

Reid, David. *The Complete Book of Chinese Health and Healing.* Boston: Shambala, 1988.

Aromatherapy

Aromatherapy Institute of Research
P.O. Box 2354
Fair Oaks, CA 95628
(916) 965-7546

National Association for Holistic Aromatherapy
P.O. Box 17622
Boulder, CO 80308
(303) 258-3791

Lotus Light
P.O. Box 1008
Wilmot, WI 53170
(414) 889-8501

READING LIST

Hymann, Daniele. *Aromatherapy: The Complete Guide to Plant and Flower Essences*. New York: Bantam Books, 1991.

Lavabre, Marcel. *Aromatherapy Workbook*. Rochester, VT: Healing Arts Press, 1990.

Rose, Jeanne. *The Aromatherapy Book*. Berkeley, CA: North Atlantic Books, 1992.

Ayurvedic Medicine

Ayurvedic Institute
11311 Menaul NE Suite A
Albuquerque, NM 87112
(505) 291-9698

Ayurvedic Rehabilitation Center
103 Bennett Street
Brighton, MA 02135

American School of Ayurvedic Sciences
10025 NE 4th Street
Bellevue, Washington 98004
(206) 453-8022

The College of Maharishi
Ayurveda Health Center
P.O. Box 282
Fairfield, IA 52556
(515) 472-5866

Maharishi Ayurveda Health Center
679 George Hill Road
P.O. Box 344
Lancaster, MA 01523

READING LIST

Chopra, Deepak, M.D. *Ageless Body, Timeless Mind.*
New York: Harmony Books, 1993. *Perfect Health*, 1991.
Quantum Healing, 1990.

David, O.M.D. *Ayurvedic Healing.* Salt Lake City: Morson
Publishing, 1990.

Heyn, Birgit. *Ayurveda: The Indian Art of Natural Medicine and
Life Extension.* Rochester, VT: Healing Arts Press, 1983.

Biofeedback

Association for Applied Psychophysiology and Biofeedback
10200 West 44th Avenue, Suite 304
Wheat Ridge, CO 80033
(303) 422-8436

Biofeedback Certification Institute of America
10200 West 44th Avenue, Suite 304
Wheat Ridge, CO 80033
(303) 420-2902

Center for Applied Psychophysiology
Menninger Clinic
P.O. Box 829
Topeka, KS 66601
(913) 273-7500

READING LIST

Danskin, David G., and Crow, Mark. *Biofeedback: An Introduction and Guide.* Palo Alto, CA: Mayfield Publishing Co., 1981.

Chiropractic

American Chiropractic Association
1701 Clarendon Boulevard
Arlington, VA 22209
(703) 276-8800

International Chiropractors Association
1110 North Glebe Road, Suite 1000
Arlington, VA 22201
(703) 528-5000

World Chiropractic Alliance
2950 N. Dobson Road, Suite 1
Chandler, AZ 85224
(800) 347-1011

READING LIST

Coplan-Griffiths, Michael. *Dynamic Chiropractic Today: The Complete and Authoritative Guide to This Major Therapy.* San Francisco: HarperCollins, 1991.

Palmer, Daniel David. *The Chiropractor's Adjuster.* Davenport, IA: Palmer College Press, 1992.

Diet and Nutrition

American College of Nutrition
722 Robert E. Lee Drive
Wilmington, North Carolina 28480
(919) 452-1222

American College of Advancement in Medicine
P.O. Box 3427
Laguna Hills, CA 92654
(714) 583-7666

READING LIST

Braverman, Eric R., M.D., and Pfeiffer, Carl C., M.D.
The Healing Nutrients Within. New Canaan, CT: Keats
Publishing, Inc., 1987.

Hass, Elson M., M.D. *Staying Healthy with Nutrition.*
Berkeley, CA: Celestial Arts Publishing, 1992.

Lappe, Frances Moore. *Diet for a Small Planet.* New York:
Ballantine, 1982.

Weil, Andrew. *Natural Health, Natural Medicine.* New York:
Houghton-Mifflin, 1990.

Heart Disease

The American Heart Association
7320 Greenville Avenue
Dallas, Texas 75231
(214) 373-6300

National Heart, Lung, and Blood Institute
National Institutes of Health
7200 Wisconsin Avenue, Suite 500
Bethesda, MD 20814
(301) 951-3260

National High Blood Pressure Education Program
Information Center
National Institutes of Health
7200 Wisconsin Avenue, Suite 500
Bethesda, MD 20814
(301) 951-3260

READING LIST

Bennet, Charles. *Controlling High Blood Pressure Without Drugs.* New York: Doubleday Books, 1984.

Cooper, Kenneth. *Overcoming Hypertension.* New York: Bantam, 1990.

Ornish, Dean, M.D. *Reversing Heart Disease.* New York: Ballantine, 1990.

Salander, James M., M.D., LeVert, Suzanne. *If It Runs in Your Family: Hypertension.* New York: Bantam Books, 1993.

Zaret, Barry L., M.D., ed. *Yale University School of Medicine Heart Book.* New York: Hearst Books, 1992.

Herbal Medicine

American Association of Naturopathic Physicians
2366 Eastlake Avenue, Suite 322
Seattle, WA 98102
(206) 323-7610

The American Botanical Council
P.O. Box 201660
Austin, TX 78720-1660
(512) 331-8868

The American Herbalists Guild
P.O. Box 1683
Sequel, CA 95073
(408) 438-1700

Herb Research Foundation
1007 Pearl Street, Suite 200
Boulder, CO 80302
(303) 449-2265

READING LIST

Castleman, Michael. *The Healing Herbs*. Emmaus, PA:
Rodale Press, 1991.

Hoffman, David. *The Herbal Handbook*. Rochester, VT:
Healing Arts Press, 1987.

Homeopathy

Homeopathic Educational Services
2124 Kittredge Street
Berkeley, CA 94704
(800) 359-9051

International Foundation for Homeopathy
2366 Eastlake Avenue
Seattle, WA 98102
(206) 324-8230

National Center for Homeopathy
801 North Fairfax
Alexandria, VA 22314
(703) 548-7790

READING LIST

Cummings, Stephen, M.D. *Everybody's Guide to Homeopathic Medicines*. Los Angeles: Jeremy P. Tarcher, Inc., 1991.

Lockie, Andrew. *The Family Guide to Homeopathy*. New York: Prentice-Hall Press, 1993.

Ullman, Dana. *Discovering Homeopathy: Medicine for the 21st Century*. North Atlantic Books, 1991.

Meditation and Mind/Body Medicine

Institute of Transpersonal Psychology
P.O. Box 4437
Stanford, CA 94305
(415) 327-2066

Mind-Body Clinic
New England Deaconess Hospital
Harvard Medical School
185 Pilgrim Road
Cambridge, MA 02215
(617) 632-9530

Stress Reduction Clinic
University of Massachusetts Medical Center
55 Lake Avenue, North
Worcester, MA 01655
(508) 856-2656

The Center for Mind-Body Studies
5225 Connecticut Avenue NW
Washington, D.C. 20015
(202) 966-7388

READING LIST

Benson, Herbert. *The Relaxation Response.* New York: Outlet
  Books, Inc., 1993.

Borysenko, Joan. *Mending the Body, Mending the Mind.* New
  York: Bantam Books, 1988.

Locke, Steven and Colligan, Douglas. *The Healer Within.* New
  York: Mentor, 1986.

Moyers, Bill. *Healing and the Mind.* New York: Doubleday, 1993.

Yoga

Himalayan Institute of Yoga, Science, and Philosophy
RRI Box 400
Honesdale, PA 18431
(800) 822-4547

International Association of Yoga Therapists
109 Hillside Avenue
Mill Valley, CA 94941
(415) 383-4587

READING LIST

Hewitt, James. *The Complete Yoga Book*. New York:
Schocken Books, 1977.

Monro, Robin, M.D., et al. *Yoga for Common Ailments*.
Fireside Books, 1990.

Alternative Medicine/General Information

American Holistic Medical Association
4101 Lake Boone Trail, Suite 201
Raleigh, NC 27607
(919) 787-5146

READING LIST

Allenburg, Henry Edward, M.D. *Holistic Medicine*. New York:
Kodansha, 1992.

Goldberg Group (350 physicians). *Alternative Medicine:
The Definitive Guide*. Puyallap, WA: Future Medicine
Publishing, Inc., 1993.

Mills, Simon, M.A., and Finando, Steven J., Ph.D. *Alternatives
in Healing*. New York: New American Library, 1988.

Monte, Tom, and editors of *EastWest Natural Health*.
*World Medicine: The East West Guide to Healing Your
Body*. New York: Tarcher/Perigree, 1993.

Murray, Michael, and Pizzorno, Joseph. *Encyclopedia of
Natural Medicine*. Rocklin, CA: Prima Publishing, 1991.

Alphabetical Directory of Cardiovascular Drug Groups

....

ACE inhibitors. Act to prevent production of a hormone, angiotensin II, that constricts blood vessels (ACE stands for angiotensin-converting enzyme). In addition to dilating blood vessels, ACE inhibitors also work to prevent the abnormal rise in hormones associated with high blood pressure and heart disease, including aldosterone, which acts on the kidneys to retain salt and water.

Special considerations: ACE inhibitors are relatively new—they were first introduced in 1981—and are quite expensive. ACE inhibitors should be avoided by anyone with impaired liver function and pregnant or breast-feeding women. Their side effects may be more severe in the elderly. They are especially useful for diabetics who have high blood pressure and/or atherosclerosis, because ACE inhibitors rarely raise glucose or blood lipid levels as do many other medications.

Possible side effects: Dizziness or weakness, loss of appetite and/or nausea, a hacking cough, and swelling.

Generic and trade names: captopril (Capoten); enalapril (Vasotec); lisinopril (Prinivil, Zestril).

Anticoagulants. Inhibit the ability of the blood to clot and prevent clots from forming or growing in blood vessels. These agents are especially useful in preventing heart attacks or strokes after heart surgery, since they prevent blood clots from forming around damaged tissue.

Special considerations: In general, anticoagulants are prescribed for just 6 to 8 months as a temporary measure following surgery or cardiovascular injury, such as stroke or heart attack. Anticoagulants interact with many other kinds of drugs, including aspirin (an antiplatelet drug, see below), oral contraceptives, and laxatives. If you are pregnant or have impaired kidney or liver function, anticoagulants may not be right for you.

Possible side effects: Excessive bleeding or bruising from minor injury; nausea and/or vomiting; and hair loss.

Generic and trade names: warfarin (Coumadin, Panwarfarin).

Antiplatelets. Like anticoagulants, work to keep blood from abnormally clotting. They act on a type of blood cell known as platelets by making them less sticky and thus less likely to clump together and clot. Antiplatelets are prescribed to prevent heart attacks and strokes in people with atherosclerosis.

Special considerations: The most common antiplatelet drug regimen is low doses of aspirin taken every day. Antiplatelets also reduce the severity and frequency of angina. They should be taken with caution by anyone with digestive system problems (such as ulcers), bleeding disorders, or who is pregnant or breast-feeding.

Possible side effects: Nausea, vomiting, or indigestion.

Generic and trade names: acetylsalicylic acid or aspirin (Alka-Selzer, Anacin, Bayer, Buffrin, Ecotrin), dipyridamole (Persantine).

Beta blockers. Work by blocking the action of the beta receptors in the heart, blood vessels, and other parts of the body. This effect stops the action of neurotransmitters that have been released by the sympathetic nervous system and thus reduces blood flow from the heart, lessens vessel action throughout the body, and blocks the production of renin—the enzyme responsible for stimulating the kidney to retain salt and water. Because these drugs relieve angina, they may be the drug of choice for people who have this problem along with high blood pressure. They are most effective when prescribed in low doses along with a diuretic.

Special considerations: Beta blockers are not recommended for people with asthma (they tend to cause spasm in the bronchial tubes) or with circulatory problems in their hands or feet.

Possible side effects: Weakness; lethargy; cold hands and feet due to reduced circulation; nausea; nightmares; and impotence.

Calcium-channel blockers. Work to relax the muscles in vessel walls by lessening the availability of calcium—a mineral that affects the rate at which muscles contract—to the cells in the arterial walls. These drugs also lessen the action of the heart muscle and are thus often used to treat angina. They can also be helpful in treating congestive heart failure.

Special considerations: Calcium-channel blockers lower blood pressure in about 30 to 40 percent of those who take them; however, they tend to be expensive and are usually prescribed only when other less expensive drugs have failed. Furthermore, recent reprints suggest that calcium-channel blockers used to lower blood pressure in asymptomatic people may increase the risk of a fatal heart attack occurring. Blacks appear to respond well to calcium-channel blockers, which also have a mild diuretic effect that relieves some of the sodium/water retention especially common among the black population.

Possible side effects: Dizziness, headache, constipation, lethargy, nausea, and swelling.

Generic and trade names: diltiazem (Cardizem), nicardipine (Cardene), nifedipine (Procardia, Procardia XL), nimodipine (Nimotop), verapamil (Calan, Isoptin, Verelan).

Diuretics. Commonly referred to as water pills, reduce the volume of the body's blood and fluids—and hence the blood pressure—by increasing the kidney's excretion of sodium and water. Treatment with diuretics causes about a 2-quart reduction in a person's fluid volume; this lower volume lessens both heart action and pressure on the vessel walls.

Special considerations: In November, 1992, the National High Blood Pressure Education Program announced that diuretics remain the most effective, and least expensive, drug to reduce high blood pressure. In addition, diuretics are the only blood pressure drugs proven to decrease the number of strokes and the incidence of heart failure among people who take them.

Today, there are three types of diuretics. The most commonly prescribed are the *thiazides*, which block the reabsorption of sodium and chloride back into the bloodstream. *Loop diuretics* are stronger drugs, usually reserved for people whose blood pressure is not adequately lowered by the thiazides or who have damaged kidneys. Loop diuretics, so named because they work in the part of the kidney known as the loop of Henle, are quite potent; in fact they eliminate about 15 percent more salt from the kidneys than do the thiazides. The third type of diuretic includes the *potassium-sparing agents*. This class of drugs was developed when physicians discovered that, along with sodium, diuretics eliminated another essential mineral, potassium. Potassium is essential for proper muscle function, and that includes heart action. When potassium loss does occur, people experience a number of dangerous side effects, including irregular heartbeat, muscle weakness, kidney malfunction, and often glucose intolerance, which may trigger or exacerbate diabetes mellitus. Potassium-sparing diuretics work in the kidneys to increase sodium excretion while maintaining potassium levels. They are usually paired with another diuretic to compensate for the potential loss of potassium.

Possible side effects: Lethargy, cramps, rash, and impotence.

Generic and trade names: chlorthalidone (Hygroton), hydrochlorothiazide (Esidrix, Hydro-Diuril, Oretic), metolazone (Diulo,

Mykrox, Zaroxolyn), bumetanide (Bumex), furosemide (Lasix), amiloride (Midamor), spironolactone (Aldactone).

Lipid-lowering drugs. Lower the amount of lipids, or fats, circulating in the blood, thereby reducing or preventing atherosclerosis. There are two main types of lipid-lowering drugs—those that act on the liver by blocking the conversion of fatty acids to lipids; and those that act to reduce the absorption of bile salts (substances containing large amounts of cholesterol that are secreted from the liver into the intestine) into the blood. Different drugs affect different parts of the patient's "total lipid profile," including high-density lipoprotein (HDL), low-density lipoprotein (LDL), and triglycerides.

Special considerations: Drugs used to lower cholesterol are prescribed *only* in combination with dietary restrictions to lower the intake of fat and cholesterol. If a person on drug therapy for high blood cholesterol continues to eat a high-fat, high-cholesterol diet, the effects of the medication may be completely undermined.

Possible side effects: Constipation, bloating, nausea, headaches, diarrhea, dizziness, rapid heartbeat, insomnia.

Generic and trade names: cholestyramine (Questran, Questran Light), colestipol (Colestid), gemfibrozil (Lopid), lovastatin (Mevacor), nicotinic acid or niacin (Nia-Bid, Niacels, Nicolar), probucol (Lorelco).

Nitrates. The oldest coronary artery medication, are potent vein and artery dilators used to treat angina pectoris. Nitrates relax the muscles surrounding the blood vessels so that they widen, thereby improving blood flow through the heart.

Special considerations: Nitrates are often the first drug of choice to treat angina, and some of these drugs interact with antihypertensive medication to lower blood pressure.

Possible side effects: Headaches, flushing, dizziness, and fainting.

Generic and trade names: nitroglycerin (Deponit NTG, Minitran, Nitro-Bid, Nitrogard, Nitroglyn, Nitrol, Nitrolingual, Nitrong, Nitrostat, Transderm-Nitro, Tridil), isosorbide dinitrate (Dilatrate-SR, Iso-Bid, Isordil, Sorbitrate, Sorbitrate SA).

Sympatholytics. Also known as alpha-adrenergic drugs, work through the sympathetic nervous system to prevent the constriction of blood vessels that causes blood pressure to rise. By doing so, they widen the blood vessels in many parts of the body. There are four different types of sympatholytics, each of which works on a different part of the body. *Central acting drugs* lower blood pressure by stimulating certain nerve receptors, located in the brain itself, which act to reduce heart rate, the amount of blood pumped by the heart, and the resistance of the blood vessels. *Peripheral inhibitors* interfere with the release of norepinephrine from sympathetic nerve endings. Without norepinephrine, vessel walls will not contract and blood pressure will not rise. *Alpha blockers* are designed to lower blood pressure by dilating the arteries and arterioles. Alpha blockers often raise the level of HDLs (the "good cholesterol") while lowering total lipid levels, which is why they are especially useful to people who suffer from both high blood pressure and coronary heart disease. *Beta blockers*, described above, are also considered sympatholytics.

Special considerations: Centrally acting drugs are not widely used in initial treatment of high blood pressure but are given along with a diuretic or other antihypertensive drug; peripheral inhibitors, although among the least expensive drugs, tend to cause drowsiness; alpha blockers are usually used in combination with other antihypertensive drugs.

Possible side effects: Orthostatic hypotension (lowering of blood pressure when a person stands up), nausea, headache, palpitation, impotence, nightmares, loss of appetite, rash, joint pains, shortness of breath.

Words and Terms to Remember

....

Active movement: Normal range of voluntary movement of a joint.

Acupoints: Acupuncture points throughout the body that correspond to specific organs.

Adrenal glands: Hormone-producing (endocrine) glands, located on top of each kidney, responsible for secreting several hormones related to the regulation of blood pressure, including epinephrine and aldosterone.

Aerobic exercise: Physical exercise that relies on oxygen for energy production.

Aldosterone: A steroid hormone that is released by the adrenal gland and acts on the kidney to promote conservation of sodium and water, thereby raising blood pressure.

Allopathy: Term for standard Western medicine; from the Greek *allos* (different) and *pathein* (disease, suffering), thus implying the use of drugs whose effects are different from those of the disease being treated.

Alpha blockers: Drugs that lower blood pressure by working with the autonomic nervous system to dilate the blood vessels.

Anaerobic exercise: Exercise that draws upon the muscles' own stores of energy and does not require oxygen, such as weight lifting and isometric exercises.

Angina: A form of heart disease involving severe pain and a feeling of pressure in the chest, often extending into the shoulder and arms.

Angiogram: A diagnostic x-ray of blood vessels or other parts of the circulatory system. The procedure involves injecting dye into the bloodstream to make blood vessels or the heart visible on an x-ray.

Anti-inflammatory: A substance that soothes inflammation or reduces the inflammatory response of the tissue directly.

Aorta: The largest artery in the body, from which all others branch; the main vessel leading away from the heart.

Arrhythmia: Irregular heartbeat.

Arteries: Blood vessels that carry blood and oxygen away from the heart to nourish cells throughout the body. The walls consist of muscle, which contracts or dilates to raise or lower blood pressure.

Arteriogram: An examination of a portion of the circulatory system performed by injecting dye through a catheter into the arteries, thereby forming a map of the blood vessels.

Atherosclerosis: A disease of the arteries in which fatty plaques develop on the inner walls.

Autonomic nervous system: The part of the nervous system responsible for bodily functions such as the heartbeat, blood pressure, and digestion. It is divided into two divisions, the sympathetic nervous system and the parasympathetic nervous system.

Beta blocker: A drug that prevents stimulation of certain receptors of the nerves of the sympathetic nervous system, which would otherwise increase the heart rate.

Biofeedback: A behavior modification therapy in which people are taught to control bodily functions such as blood pressure through conscious effort.

Blood: In Chinese medicine, the most dense fluid substance in the body, which provides the essence in which the intellect and the emotions "live."

Blood pressure: The force exerted by blood as it is pumped by the heart and presses against the blood vessel walls.

Calcium-channel blockers: Drugs that keep some calcium from reaching the smooth muscle of the blood vessels, thereby dilating the vessels and lowering arterial pressure.

Carbohydrate: Organic compounds of carbon, hydrogen, and oxygen, which include starches, cellulose, and sugars, and an important source of energy. All carbohydrates are eventually broken down in the body to glucose, a simple sugar.

Cardiovascular system: The heart together with the two networks of blood vessels (veins and arteries) that transport nutrients and oxygen to the tissues and remove waste products.

Carminative: Term in herbal medicine to denote plants that help the digestive system to work properly by soothing any inflammation that might be present and removing any excess gas in the digestive tract.

Catheterization: A procedure in which a small flexible tube is inserted into the body in the process of diagnosis or treatment, as in an arteriogram.

Central nervous system: The brain and the spinal cord, which are responsible for the integration of all neurological functions.

Channels: Also called meridians; in traditional Chinese medicine, the invisible pathways of qi both on the surface of and within the body.

Chinese medicine: A philosophy and methodology of health and medicine developed in ancient China.

Cholesterol: A fatlike substance found in the brain, nerves, liver, blood, and bile. Synthesized in the liver, cholesterol is essential in a number of bodily functions.

Coronary arteries: The two vessels coming from the aorta to the heart. They go on to branch and supply the heart muscle with blood.

Coronary artery disease: Disease of the heart caused by a narrowing of the coronary arteries, resulting in reduced blood flow to the heart.

Detoxification: In Ayurveda, the process of removing toxins from the body.

Diastole: The interval between heartbeats when the heart relaxes and fills with blood. The diastolic reading in a blood pressure measurement is the lower number.

Diuretic: Any substance—natural or pharmaceutical—that works to lower the volume of the blood by promoting salt and water excretion by the way of the urine.

Doshas: In Ayurvedic medicine, the three basic biological types which determine an individual's constitution.

Echocardiography: Diagnostic procedure that uses ultrasound waves to visualize structures within the heart.

Electrocardiography (ECG or EKG): A procedure in which heart function is measured by the tracing of its electrical impulses.

Endocrine system: A network of glands that secrete hormones into the bloodstream. Hormones help to control body processes including digestion, circulation, reproduction, and growth

Endorphins: Natural substances produced by the body which function as natural painkillers.

Epinephrine: Also called adrenaline. A hormone secreted by the adrenal glands that increases the heart rate and constricts blood vessels.

Essential fatty acids: Unsaturated fatty acids which cannot be synthesized in the body and are considered essential for maintaining health.

Essential oil: Concentrated, pure aromatic essence extracted from plants.

Excess condition: In traditional Chinese medicine, a condition in which qi, blood, or body fluids are disordered and accumulate in channels or elsewhere in the body.

Fat: An essential nutrient, the principal form in which energy is stored in the body.

Fight-or-flight response: The body's response to perceived danger or stress, involving the release of hormones and subsequent rise in heart rate, blood pressure, and muscle tension.

Five Phases theory: In Chinese medicine, a way of looking at the body and the universe that explains the interaction between them.

Free radicals: Molecules that are highly reactive and potentially destructive to the body.

Glucose: The most common simple sugar; essential source of energy for the body.

Heart attack: Also called myocardial infarction. Death of heart tissue caused by an interruption of the blood circulation through the coronary arteries.

Heart rate: The number of times the heart beats (contracts and releases) each minute.

Hemoglobin: The oxygen-carrying red pigment component of the red blood cells. Hemoglobin transports oxygen to the body tissue and removes carbon dioxide.

High-density lipoprotein: A lipid-carrying protein, also known as the "good cholesterol," associated with a reduced risk of atherosclerosis.

Holistic: Pertaining to the whole body; treatment of disease by taking into consideration every part of the body, not only the presenting symptoms, to bring the internal environment into balance.

Homeopathic remedy: A remedy, selected on the basis of the similarity of its symptoms, that produces a reaction in a patient that stimulates an immune system response.

Hormone: Internal secretion that is transported by the bloodstream to various organs to regulate or modify vital bodily functions and processes.

Hyperlipidemia: Excessive fats in the blood.

Hypertension: High blood pressure.

Infarction: The death of tissue that occurs when the blood supply to a localized part of the body is blocked.

Insulin: A hormone produced and secreted by the pancreas; necessary for proper metabolism, particularly of carbohydrates and the uptake of glucose.

Ischemia: Oxygen deficiency caused by an obstruction of a blood vessel.

Kidneys: The two bean-shaped glands, situated at the back of the abdomen, that regulate salt volume and composition of the body fluids by filtering the blood and eliminating waste through the production of urine.

Law of Similars: The principle that "like shall be cured by like" that forms the basis of homeopathy; the proper remedy for a patient's disease is that substance that is capable of producing, in a healthy person, symptoms similar to those from which the patient suffers.

Limbic system: A group of brain structures that influence the endocrine and autonomic nervous systems.

Lipids: Fats, steroids, phospholipids, and glycolipids; fat or fatlike substances.

Low-density lipoprotein: The lipid-carrying protein, also known as the "bad cholesterol," associated with an increased risk of atherosclerosis.

Manipulation: Technique used in chiropractic therapy to adjust the spine, joints, and other tissue.

Meridians: In traditional Chinese medicine, the fourteen channels in the body through which qi runs.

Methionine: An essential amino acid.

Mobilization: A technique of chiropractic therapy that gently increases the range of movement of a joint.

Moxa: Dried mugwort leaves used in traditional Chinese medicine; placed on the end of needles, then lighted and held near an acupuncture point to warm and tonify qi.

Musculoskeletal system: Pertaining to the muscles and skeleton.

Neurotransmitters: Substances that transmit messages to, from, and within the brain and other body tissues.

Nicotine: A chemical substance derived from tobacco that affects blood pressure and pulse rate.

Norepinephrine: A hormone secreted by the adrenal gland that raises blood pressure by constricting small blood vessels and increasing blood flow through the coronary arteries.

Obesity: The condition in which excess fat has accumulated in the body; usually considered to be present when a person is 20 percent above the recommended weight for his or her height.

Oxygenation: To supply or combine with oxygen.

Palpation: Physical examination of the body using hands to feel for abnormalities.

Pancreas: The gland situated behind the stomach that secretes a number of substances important for digestion, including the hormone insulin.

Parasympathetic nervous system: The division of the nervous system that, when stimulated, slows heart rate, lowers blood pressure, and slows breathing.

Pitta: An Ayurvedic dosha.

Plaque: Fatty deposits that build up on the inner walls of the blood vessels, resulting in obstruction of the normal flow of blood.

Platelet: Component of the blood involved in blood clotting.

Potency: The dilution of homeopathic remedies to increase their effectiveness, thus giving them their therapeutic value.

Qi: In traditional Chinese medicine, the life-force or energy of the body and the universe that circulates through the body's channels.

Qi stagnation: Any blockage of energy in the body that interrupts the body's natural functions or the healing process.

Risk factor: Condition or behavior that increases one's likelihood of developing a disease or injury.

Saturated fat: Type of fat derived mainly from animal products associated with an elevation of blood cholesterol levels and atherosclerosis.

Sclerosis: An abnormal thickening or hardening of the arteries and other vessels.

Shen: In traditional Chinese medicine, the "spirit" or consciousness, which both originates and forms the outward expression of human life.

Stress: Any factor, physical or emotional, that provokes a physical response, positive or negative, in the body.

Stroke: An interruption of the blood flow to the brain causing damage and loss of function.

Subluxation: In chiropractic, a term used to explain a misalignment of spinal vertebrae.

Succussion: The forceful shaking of liquid homeopathic remedies that allows the permeation of the medicinal substance into the alcohol tincture.

Sympathetic nervous system: The division of the autonomic nervous system responsible for such actions as blood pressure, salivation, and digestion; works in balance with the parasympathetic nervous system.

Symptoms: Observable or internal changes in the mental, emotional, and physical condition of a person; in holistic medicine, symptoms are the external proof of an internal imbalance.

Systole: The contraction of the heart muscle; systolic pressure is the greater of the two numbers in a blood pressure reading.

Tao: The course of nature and ways of nature; a Chinese term denoting the universe as an undifferentiated whole.

Thrombosis: The formation of a blood clot, called a thrombus, that partially or completely blocks a blood vessel.

Tincture: An alcoholic solution of a medicinal substance.

Tonify: In Chinese medicine, to nourish, augment, and invigorate; to add to the supply of qi and to promote the proper functioning and balance in the body.

Toxin: Substance that is harmful or poisonous to the body.

Transient ischemic attack (TIA): An interruption of blood supply to a part of the brain that causes temporary impairment of vision, speech, or movement.

Triglyceride: The most common lipid found in fatty tissue; the form in which fat is stored in the body.

Vascular: Pertaining to or supplied with blood vessels.

Vasoconstrictor: An agent that causes blood vessels to narrow, thereby causing a decrease in blood flow.

Vasodilator: An agent that causes the blood vessels to widen, thereby increasing blood flow.

Vata: An Ayurvedic dosha.

Vital force: In homeopathy, the intangible energy that animates all living creatures and mediates their physical, emotional, and intellectual responses to external stress.

Yang organs: In Chinese medicine, the yang organs include the intestines, gallbladder, and skin.

Yin organs: In Chinese medicine, the yin organs are dense, internal organs such as the heart, liver, lungs, kidneys, and bones.

Yin/Yang: Chinese concept that describes all existence in terms of states or conditions that are different but mutually dependent; traditional Chinese medicine aims to restore balance to these contrasting aspects of the body and mind.

Index

About the Authors

Glenn S. Rothfeld, M.D.

Glenn S. Rothfeld, M.D., is founder and Medical Director of Spectrum Medical Arts in Arlington, Massachusetts, a comprehensive primary care center blending orthodox and complementary medical styles. He holds one of the nation's first Master's Degrees in acupuncture, and is director of Western Medical Curriculum at the New England School of Acupuncture. He is also Clinical Instructor at Tufts University School of Medicine, where he teaches a popular course in Natural Medicine.

Suzanne LeVert

Suzanne LeVert is a writer who specializes in health and medical subjects. Her recent titles include A Woman Doctor's Guide to Menopause, Parkinson's Disease: A Complete Guide for Patients and Caregivers, *and* If It Runs in the Family: Hypertension and Diabetes. *She lives in Boston, Massachusetts.*